Alzheimer's Disease and Dementia in Down Syndrome and Intellectual Disabilities

Vee P Prasher
Consultant Neuro-Psychiatrist
South Birmingham Primary Care Trust
and
Senior Research Fellow
King's College London

Foreword by
Matthew P Janicki

Radcliffe Publishing
Oxford • Seattle

Radcliffe Publishing Ltd
18 Marcham Road
Abingdon
Oxon OX14 1AA
United Kingdom

www.radcliffe-oxford.com
Electronic catalogue and worldwide online ordering facility.

British Library Cataloguing in Publication Data

A catalogue record for this book is available from the British Library.

ISBN 1 85775 608 8

Typeset by Anne Joshua & Associates, Oxford
Printed and bound by TJ International Ltd, Padstow, Cornwall

To Professor John Corbett, former Professor of Developmental Psychiatry, University of Birmingham, who inspired myself and so many others to work with people with intellectual disability

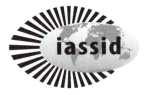

This book is endorsed by the IASSID

Contents

Foreword

There has been a dramatic shift in the awareness and concern over lifespan challenges facing people with intellectual disabilities worldwide. Much of this awakening can be attributed to both general population aging in the developed world and a greater recognition that people with a range of intellectual disabilities, too, are surviving in greater numbers into old age. Yet, as health authorities and practitioners gear up to accommodate a range of normal health issues among the increasing number of older people, they too are becoming more aware of a variety of age-associated and age-related pathological conditions that have become more pronounced among aging people. One area of worldwide concern is the expected dramatic increase in the prevalence of Alzheimer's disease, due to the expected growth in the absolute number of people surviving into old age.

With this text, Vee Prasher, one of the most prominent authorities on age-related conditions among people with intellectual disabilities, and in particular Alzheimer's disease, has tackled a topic that is beginning to vigorously emerge within the intellectual disabilities field. Much has happened over the past quarter century to move considerations of the needs and condition of people with intellectual disabilities from simplistic formulations and debates over the proper place of housing to a sophisticated and highly nuanced exploration of needs, wants, and health and social conditions that mirror those of the general population. One of these emerging concerns is what happens when lifelong disability combines with the organic nature of aging. In many instances, the knowledge and technology emanating from the fields of gerontology and geriatrics are helping us to better understand the possibilities and expectations for aging when combined with primary lifelong conditions. When health compromises have been the norm over a lifetime then more is known about the limitations on extended longevity and the emergence of probable secondary conditions. With Down syndrome, enough research is now extant that we know in many instances adults who enter their late middle age are at high probable risk for the occurrence of Alzheimer's disease and the resulting emergence of Alzheimer's related dementia. Now that the extensive research and practice knowledge around this issue has been assembled and synthesized into one comprehensive text – as has been done here – this information can be presented and put to use in a range of clinical practice situations.

The field of intellectual disabilities has come a long way since those dark days when institutionalization was the norm and the published research dwelt on the dysfunctional and devalued character of the people in those settings. While some pioneers began to explore the age-associated effects of longevity among people with Down syndrome, these explorations were more in the vein of clinical descriptives and not prescriptives. In the intervening years, the changing beliefs and philosophical underpinnings of services for people with ID has forced a change in orientation from simply identifying problems to defining and articulating a wide range of solutions and potential avenues for living constructive lives and self-determination. The area of age-associated conditions is a good example of this sea-change in orientation. In this text Vee Prasher has assembled a wealth of information that will not only permit clinicians, but families and public policy-makers as well, to appreciate that early identification and intervention when Alzheimer's is first suspected can go far towards mitigating the devastating consequences of this disease, and help specialist services focus on maintaining quality of life and enhancing practices that will help people so affected maintain their dignity until the end.

As a tool well suited for this purpose, *Alzheimer's Disease and Dementia in Down Syndrome and Intellectual Disabilities* will be a welcome addition to the growing body of literature on this disease and should provide readers with the means to more effectively prepare and respond to the nuances associated with its occurrence and progression.

Matthew P Janicki, PhD
University of Illinois at Chicago
September 2005

Preface

This book brings together findings from research and clinical practice with a multi-disciplinary perspective regarding the practical aspects of dementia care for older adults with intellectual disability, particularly adults with Down syndrome. It is most important for professionals to have a complete understanding of dementia in order to comprehend the significant aspects of research and clinical practice. Academic books can often lose the vision of a person-centred approach. Clinical practitioners, on the other hand, may not always have the most up-to-date relevant knowledge to provide the appropriate care. This book aims to fill that gap.

In addition, the significant research and clinical aspects of Alzheimer's disease in the general population are discussed and put in relevant context for adults with intellectual disability. Undoubtedly research and clinical practice are much more advanced in the general population than in adults with intellectual disability. It is therefore important that professionals and academics in the field of intellectual disability are made fully aware of ongoing developments in the general population which will very probably become important to the intellectually disabled population. This book is the first to incorporate factual information on Alzheimer's disease and its associated dementia in the general population with that for adults with intellectual disability.

Dementia in the intellectually disabled population cannot be discussed merely as a disease entity *per se*. The impact on the person him- or herself and on his or her carers always needs to be taken into account. Caring for intellectually disabled adults who develop dementia requires a multi-disciplinary approach. Services require further development, and carers should have a greater say in the future development of specialist homes for intellectually disabled adults with dementia, in the development of tertiary services (such as memory clinics) and in determining future areas of research.

The term *intellectual disabilities* has been used throughout this book. The term has yet to gain universal acceptance, and the author is aware that other terms with a similar meaning are used across the world. For example, the terms *mental retardation*, *learning disabilities*, *mental handicap*, *developmental disability* and *intellectual handicap* (or variants of these) are used in other nations. In this book the term *intellectual disabilities* is considered to be synonymous with these other terms.

The basic aim of this book is to help carers and professionals who are living or working with adults with intellectual disability to increase their understanding of Alzheimer's disease and other forms of dementia. This volume aims to put research into clinical practice and if, as a result, one person with intellectual disability has their dementia diagnosed early, treated appropriately and professionally and their carers are supported with sympathy and compassion, the book will not have been published in vain.

Vee Prasher
September 2005
vprasher@compuserve.com

Acknowledgements

I wish to thank each individual with Down syndrome and their families who allowed me to spend time with them over the last 15 years and to use their photographs. I am also grateful to Lesley Seeney, my secretary, who patiently helped with early drafts of this book, to Janette Hill, librarian, who over many years helped to collect many of the research papers, and to Dr Peter Barber, Dr Martyn Carey and Dr Ted Rolfe, who provided the neuropathological and neuroimaging photographs.

List of abbreviations

AChE	acetylcholinesterase
AD	Alzheimer's disease
ApoE	apolipoprotein E
APP	amyloid precursor protein
CJD	Creutzfeldt–Jakob disease
CT	computerised tomography
DAD	dementia in Alzheimer's disease
DMR	Dementia Questionnaire for Mentally Retarded Persons
DS	Down syndrome
DSDS	Down Syndrome Dementia Scale
DSM-IV	*Diagnostic and Statistical Manual of Mental Disorders – Fourth Edition*
EEG	electroencephalography
HIV	human immunodeficiency virus
ICD-9	*International Classification of Diseases and Related Health Problems – Ninth Revision*
ICD-10	*International Classification of Diseases and Related Health Problems – Tenth Revision*
ID	intellectual disabilities
MDT	multi-disciplinary team
MMSE	Mini Mental State Examination
MRI	magnetic resonance imaging
NSF	National Service Framework
PET	positron emission tomography
PS1	presenilin 1
PS2	presenilin 2
SPECT	single photon emission computed tomography
VEP	visual evoked potential

List of plates

Chapter 1

Overview of dementia in intellectual disabilities

Introduction

During the last quarter of the twentieth century, providers of health and social care have become acutely aware of the unmet needs of the ageing general population. This has in part been due to the dramatic increase in the number of people aged 65 years and over. In the USA in 1950, 8% of the population was over the age of 65 years. By 1978 this figure had risen to 11%, and it is estimated that by the year 2030 this figure will increase to 20% (over 50 million individuals) (Schoenberg 1986). Although for the population of individuals with intellectual disabilities (ID) there has not been such a dramatic rise in the ageing population, nevertheless there has been a mirroring in the rate of increase in older adults with ID. Between the years 1990 and 2010 the number of people with Down syndrome (DS) over the age of 40 years is expected to increase by 75%, and it has been reported that the number of people with DS over the age of 50 years will increase by 200% (Steffelaar and Evenhuis 1989). At the start of the twenty-first century it is now expected that as people with ID are living longer, many will survive to their seventh or eighth decade of life and become recognised members of the community. The average life expectancy has increased not only for the general population, but also for people with ID, especially those with DS. For example, life expectancy for children with DS was reported to be approximately 9 years in 1929 (Penrose 1949), approximately 12–15 years by 1947 (Penrose 1949), 18 years in 1961 (Collman and Stoller 1963) and 57 years in 1989 (Baird and Sadovnick 1989). A life-table listing findings for 1341 individuals with DS born in British Columbia, Canada between 1952 and 1981 is shown in Table 1.1. It demonstrates that a person with DS born at the present time in the developed world can expect to survive, on average, into their fifth decade of life.

There are a number of reasons why people with ID are living longer. Principally it is because of the relative decrease in newborn and infant mortality rather than a significant increase in longevity. There have been considerable advances in infant healthcare, such as surgical intervention for congenital abnormalities, improved medical treatment for childhood infections and ongoing improvements in nutrition and health promotion. Such factors have led to a marked reduction in the mortality of infants with ID. A general increase in the standard of living, an increased awareness of prevention of health disorders by screening and improved education have all improved the longevity of people with ID. However, there is still a need for further improvements in healthcare provision, as the age-specific mortality rates do remain significantly higher for people with ID than for equivalent age groups in the general population.

Table 1.1 Life expectancy for individuals with DS

Age (years)	Survival at start of age interval (%)
0	100.00
1	87.83
2	83.92
3	82.20
4	81.44
5	81.05
10	78.40
20	75.34
30	72.12
40	69.78
50	60.68
51	60.68
52	59.53
53	56.91
54	55.49
55	53.90
60	44.44
61	38.71
62	29.03
63	29.03
64	29.03
65	24.88
66	20.36
67	13.57
68	13.57

This table is based on the original that appeared as table 5.1, pp. 49–50 in Sadovnick AD and Baird PA (1992) Life expectancy. In: Pueschel SM and Pueschel JK (eds) *Biomedical Concerns in Persons with Down Syndrome.* Paul H Brookes Publishing Co., Baltimore, MD.

The increasing size of the ageing ID population requires a corresponding increase in the allocation of resources, which has been highlighted as a potential crisis in the human service system (Jacobson and Janicki 1985). The shift in the age distribution has been compounded by the moving into 'community care' of people with ID who previously would have lived in institutions of one type or another. Until the latter half of the twentieth century, few older adults with ID were encountered in society, and healthcare professionals routinely cared for children and adults with ID in long-stay institutions with little access to community facilities.

Furthermore, clinicians are now aware that particular groups, such as people with DS, are susceptible to 'triple jeopardy'. This is when a person with DS has ID, can suffer from premature ageing, and as they grow older are also susceptible to the neuropathological changes of Alzheimer's disease (AD) and its associated clinical presentation, termed *dementia in Alzheimer's disease (DAD)*. Sadly, elderly people with ID can be further disadvantaged compared with their general population peers, as by middle and old age they are more susceptible to the death of parents and friends, have a greater susceptibility to physical health problems, and have poor access to recreational activities.

The many and varied life experiences of older people with ID have yet to be fully appreciated. Appropriate health and social services have not yet been developed to cater for the subsequent impact and effects. Experiences in particular relate to health problems, daytime occupation, living with ageing parents, living with other ageing individuals and the emotional distress associated with losses that occur in later life. None of these areas of life experience are independent of each other, but rather they overlap to a certain extent and impact on each other. This is exemplified by the onset of dementia, which has a considerable impact on an individual's health, their ability to continue to live in their present placement and their ability to relate to other individuals, and can lead to considerable carer stress associated with looking after someone with dementia. Ageing people with ID have now (and not before time) become the focus of considerable debate.

Historical background to dementia and ID

The vast majority of information on dementia and ID relates to adults with DS. The first scientifically accepted association between DS and DAD was reported by Fraser and Mitchell in 1876. Commenting on people with DS, they stated that 'in not a few instances, however, death is attributed to nothing more than general decay . . . precipitated senility'. A further 50 years elapsed before Struwe (1929) and later Bertrand and Koffas (1946) described the characteristic senile plaques (also known as amyloid or neuritic plaques) of AD in the brains of individuals with DS. In 1946, Rollin noticed the similarity between regression in DS and catatonic schizophrenia, and speculated about the decline in skills associated with the clinical condition. A definitive link between DS and the clinical and neuropathological manifestations of AD was finally described by Jervis in 1948 and confirmed by Verhaart and Jelgersma in 1952. Jervis (1948), in his paper describing three individuals with DS, aged 37, 42 and 47 years, commented that people with DS 'who reach the fourth or fifth decade of life undergo remarkable personality changes, resulting from intellectual and emotional deterioration. In these patients, the underlying brain lesions are those of pathological senility'. Subsequently, several independent researchers confirmed that virtually all adults with DS over the age of 40 years show pathological changes of AD (Malamud 1966; Wisniewski *et al.* 1985; Mann 1988), and such changes have been shown to be present in young persons with DS. Mann (1988) reviewed previously published data and investigated the presence of senile plaques and neurofibrillary tangles in the brains of individuals with DS. In a total of 34 studies, 392 patients (age range 10–79 years) were studied and, of these, 223 patients demonstrated AD changes. Of the 183 patients over 40 years of age, 180 (98.4%) had senile plaques and neurofibrillary tangles, whereas only 43 of 209 patients (20.6%) under the age of 40 years showed such changes. More recent research suggests that there are differential types of senile plaques, where some forms may be age-related and non-pathological while others are associated with the clinical features of AD (Schupf and Sergievsky 2002).

At the same time as neuropathological reports were being published, case reports and subsequently cohort studies were also being published, highlighting the clinical picture of dementia in older adults (for reviews see Oliver and Holland 1986; Prasher and Krishnan 1993; Hutchinson 1999). A characteristic picture of memory decline, intellectual deficits, loss of adaptive skills and physical problems was described, which was not too dissimilar to that seen in the general population. The most recent research studies have looked at drug therapies for DAD in adults with DS (Prasher 2004) or are investigating the prevention of the onset of DAD (Dalton *et al*, 2004).

Genetic factors and DAD

In 1959, Lejeune and his colleagues confirmed that DS was a consequence of a genetic abnormality involving triplication of chromosome 21, and did not have a racial aetiology as originally postulated by Langdon Down (Down 1862). This landmark finding subsequently led to the search for a specific gene on chromosome 21 that produced amyloid precursor protein (APP), which was known to be the principal protein associated with AD. The protein substance 'amyloid' found in the centre of the senile plaques was formed from this much larger APP fragment (Glenner and Wong 1984).

The APP gene was identified by Kang *et al.* (1987), and was located within the 21q21 band on the long arm of chromosome 21, near the critical region for DS. It was postulated that due to the triplication of chromosome 21, three APP genes were present in individuals with DS. This triplication led to overactivity of the APP gene, resulting in increased production of APP. Increased circulating levels of APP in turn led to increased deposition of amyloid and resulted in clinical dementia. Further evidence for this hypothesis comes from mutations in the APP gene leading to familial early-onset DAD (Goate *et al.* 1991), and from a case report of a person with DS who did not have triplication of the APP gene but lived to the age of 78 years without evidence of clinical or neuropathological AD (Prasher *et al.* 1998).

However, this is a considerable over-simplification, and there are other genes which may or do play a role in the development of DAD in adults with – and indeed without – DS. Recently the genotype of apolipoprotein E, which occurs in several forms, has been shown to be a strong risk factor for DAD in the general population (Roses 1994), and has been demonstrated to play a lesser role in the DS population (Deb *et al.* 2000). Superoxide dismutase 1 is an important enzyme that is needed for antioxidant defence and is localised on chromosome 21 (Anneren and Edman 1993). Enzymatic activity of superoxide dismutase 1 is elevated in people with DS, and could exert harmful effects by causing an increase in hydrogen peroxide levels. At present the role of superoxide dismutase 1 in the aetiology of AD is still unclear, but it remains an important factor. Additional factors to be considered include other as yet unidentified genes, the effect of family history of DAD, the role of premature ageing and environmental factors.

Clinico-pathological correlation

Although an association between the neuropathology of AD and DS has been established, the precise link between the two is not yet fully understood. As mentioned previously, virtually all adults with DS over the age of 40 years show marked neuropathological changes of AD in their brain tissue. This is in contrast to the general population, in whom such changes at this age are extremely rare. Research findings suggest that the clinical prevalence of DAD in adults with DS is 9% for the age range 40–49 years, 36% for the age range 50–59 years and 55% for the age range 60–69 years (Prasher 1995a). Clinical dementia is therefore not inevitable in older adults with DS who exhibit the neuropathology of AD. Dementia has been diagnosed in adults with DS as young as 30 years of age, but adults with DS have survived to over 70 years without evidence of dementia.

A number of hypotheses have been put forward to explain these inconsistent findings.

1 When the neuropathology of AD is present, clinical dementia is also present, but due to the underlying severity of ID clinicians are unable to detect clinical changes typical of dementia. If a person is already functioning at a low intellectual level they may not have the capacity to show further impairment of skills (a prerequisite for a diagnosis of dementia) – the so-called 'floor effect'. Further clinical signs and symptoms of DAD, particularly in the early stages, may be difficult to detect in older adults with DS because of the underlying severity of ID, the level of communication, phenotypic characteristics, the presence of sensory impairment (of hearing and vision), and the effects of psychotropic medication and institutionalisation. In the author's view this is an unlikely explanation for the inconsistency between neuropathological and clinical AD. Many individuals with DS show neuropathological changes of AD in their brain tissue for 20, 30 or indeed up to 50 years. It is unlikely that clinical dementia would not have been detected and diagnosed over such a time period, even allowing for the lack of accurate tests.

2 People with DS are susceptible to the characteristic neuropathological changes in the brain, but are resistant to the day-to-day clinical presentation of dementia. This hypothesis remains plausible but unlikely. One would expect that if 'disease' changes (plaques and tangles) were present for a number of decades (in all DS adults by the age of 40 years) then within a few years clinical features should be manifested. Furthermore, as people with DS already have underlying biochemical pathology due to their ID, arguably, clinical features should be seen quite early on.

3 At least two types of neuropathological changes of AD are seen in the DS population (non-pathological and pathological changes). The former are present in children and younger adults and do not lead to clinical DAD. The latter are age-related, as in the general population, occur in later life (50 years of age or over) and are associated with clinical dementia.

Summary

As demonstrated by the proliferation of published articles on this subject, the association between DS and AD is generating considerable clinical and scientific interest. However, the precise mechanisms of aetiology, the clinico-neuropatho-logical link and effective treatment strategies have yet to be fully defined. As people with ID continue to live longer, they are susceptible to age-related health disorders, especially DAD. It is important that the primary care services, particularly general practitioners, who may be the first port of call have at least a basic awareness of ageing issues in people with ID, so that they are able to direct individuals to the appropriate secondary and indeed tertiary services. Paid carers or family carers also need to be educated and made aware of health issues in older people, in particular so that these carers are able to detect symptoms that highlight the need for a medical consultation. At present few services (either health or social) have been specifically developed for older adults with ID, in particular for people with dementia. It is important that awareness of the association discussed in this chapter is instilled throughout the health service to enable specific high-quality services to be developed. The education and training of carers is also an important area.

Although this book will focus in particular on DAD in adults with DS, a number of the issues that will be discussed relate to dementia generally, and apply to all individuals with ID.

Endnote

The terms 'old' and 'elderly' have not been fully defined for people with ID. It is generally agreed that the cut-off point should be much lower than the age of 65 years which is used for the general population. Historically, a number of cut-off points have been proposed, ranging from 40 to 50 years, to retaining the statutory age of 65 years. Adults with DS are reported to age prematurely, which would support the view that for the ID population a lower cut-off point for age should be used. Although there is no definitive international consensus, a cut-off point of 55 years is widely used.

Chapter 2

Definition, classification and aetiology of dementia

What is dementia?

The outdated and inappropriate term 'senile' is sometimes still used to describe confusion in an elderly person. It is also used to imply 'someone getting old' or an elderly person who has dementia, or it may be used as a lay term for Alzheimer's disease. The term is therefore quite misleading, and should no longer be used. Instead, the more unambiguous and appropriate terms *dementia, dementia in Alzheimer's disease (DAD), Alzheimer's disease (AD)* or *age-associated cognitive decline* should be used.

The term 'dementia' is a general term used to describe a number of different disease processes and disorders with a wide range of underlying causes that lead to progressive deterioration in intellectual functioning. The commonest type of dementia is DAD (World Health Organization 1992). The World Health Organization defines dementia as 'a syndrome due to disease of the brain, usually of a chronic or progressive nature, in which there is disturbance of higher quarter functions, including memory, thinking, orientation, comprehension, calculation, learning capacity, language and judgement' (World Health Organization 1992). Consciousness is usually unimpaired in terms of a person feeling drowsy or having a fluctuating level of alertness. Impairment of cognitive function as defined above is commonly accompanied by deterioration in social skills and behaviour, and changes in emotion and motivation. It must always be borne in mind that no two people with dementia will present in exactly the same way, as their underlying personality, the severity of ID, their social and cultural background, the cause of the dementia and their physical health status are important factors in determining the clinical presentation.

However, the one characteristic symptom is the progressive and severe loss of memory. Short-term memory is particularly affected in people who have dementia. This presents as individuals forgetting things that they have just said or done, even though they can often recall quite clearly events that may have occurred many years or decades previously. It is not uncommon for carers to say 'his memory for things in the past remains good, but he just can't remember what he did a few minutes ago'. In the early stages, as well as evidence of forgetfulness, a sense of confusion with regard to time and recognition of place, and difficulty in recalling and finding words may often be apparent. A marked change in the person's personality is often reported. Some individuals who were easygoing and placid before the onset of the illness may become more irritable, aggressive and hostile. Others may become more amenable and sweet-natured. Indeed changes in personality may be more evident than memory loss, and it is documented in the literature that a person may present with 'behavioural problems' several years before a diagnosis of DAD is made. This decline in intellectual level of functioning inevitably has an impact on their everyday skills (e.g. washing, dressing, feeding), which also then deteriorate. Difficulty in communication occurs in both understanding others and making themselves understood. Behavioural problems can be quite severe, along with a number of physical problems, such as the onset of seizures (myoclonic or grand mal), incontinence and immobility. Paranoid ideas (a fixed false belief that one is being persecuted) and hallucinations (the experience of seeing or hearing something which is not present in reality) are reported to occur.

The impact of the intellectual functional decline and its interference with day-to-day and personal activities will depend on several factors, such as the underlying level of severity of the ID, whether the person has been cared for in the community or in a institution, and whether they are currently living independently or in a care facility. The social and cultural settings will therefore determine the degree, severity and subsequent impact of the intellectual functional decline on adaptive skills. In the general population, dementia may have a significant impact on an individual's ability to undertake employment. This is not a particular issue for people with ID, but nevertheless dementia can and will have an impact on their ability to perform activities at educational centres, day centres and other such places.

The different types of dementia

There are several classification systems for categorising the different types of dementia. These include classification by cause, anatomical location, course and prognosis. Box 2.1 lists some of the common types of dementia.

Box 2.1 Common types of dementia

Alzheimer's disease – associated with DS, family history
Vascular dementia – associated with hypertension, diabetes
Mixed dementia – Alzheimer's disease and vascular changes occurring together
Frontotemporal dementia
Dementia with Lewy bodies
Dementia in Pick's disease – associated with frontal lobe features
Dementia in Huntington's disease – associated with Huntington's disease
Parkinson disease dementia – seen in adults with Parkinson's disease
Alcohol-related dementia – seen in adults with chronic alcohol abuse
HIV dementia – consequence of human immunodeficiency virus (HIV) disease

---

Dementia in Alzheimer's disease (DAD)

The characteristic clinical features of DAD as seen in adults with DS are described in Chapter 4. Here a general discussion of DAD will be given.

Dementia in Alzheimer's disease came to the attention of the scientific community in 1907 when Alois Alzheimer, a German neuropathologist, described a 51-year-old woman who developed progressive symptoms of intellectual decline, particularly associated with loss of memory, disorientation, disturbance of speech and language skills, and paranoid ideas. She died a few years later, but samples of her brain were examined microscopically using several neuropathological stains, and it was found that there were numerous diffused deposits, and intensely staining neurofibrillary substances throughout the brain, subsequently termed *senile plaques* and *neurofibrillary tangles*, respectively (*see* 1 and 2, colour plate section). In recognition of the scientific contribution made by Alois Alzheimer, this disease was named *Alzheimer's disease* – that is, a specific form of dementia with the characteristic brain pathology of excess senile plaques and neurofibrillary tangles. However, 10–20% of healthy older adults in the general population may have occasional plaques and tangles, and also such pathology may be absent in 16–30% of individuals with a clinical diagnosis of DAD.

Alzheimer's disease is a disease of the brain that particularly affects the temporal regions. There is a characteristic slow progressive loss of intellectual function with associated social, behavioural and physical changes, typically lasting for between 5 and 20 years. Early death results from end-stage dementia. Dementia in Alzheimer's disease has been classified as having either early onset (before 65 years of age) or late onset (after 65 years of age), but this cut-off point is arbitrary as DAD is a continuum disorder. Early onset in the general population accounts for approximately 5–10% of cases of DAD, is often familial (i.e. there is a strong family history) and is usually associated with a chromosomal gene abnormality.

Neuropathologically there is atrophy (involving 13–18% loss of brain volume) of the cerebral hemispheres, which become shrunken and lose weight (7.5–18%) (*see* 3 and 4, colour plate section). Such a change can be seen on computed tomography (CT) or magnetic resonance imaging (MRI) scans. However, shrinkage of the cerebral hemispheres can be seen in older adults who show no evidence of dementia, so this change is not specific to AD. The shrinkage is due to loss of normal nerve cells throughout the brain, principally in the outer layer of the brain, but also in the internal structures. Research studies have shown that certain areas of the brain are susceptible to this damage, especially the temporal lobes (22–40% loss of brain cells) and the hippocampal region (43–57% loss of brain cells), an area specifically related to short-term memory. Other areas such as the frontal lobe (25–60% loss) can also be affected. As if to compensate for the loss in brain matter, there is dilatation of the ventricular fluid system within the brain, which then can increase by between a third and a half.

Microscopically the characteristic changes of senile plaques and neurofibrillary tangles can be seen in abundance (Braak and Braak 1991). Senile plaques are areas of degeneration in the brain associated with a central core protein known as beta-amyloid protein (*see* 1, colour plate section). This protein is formed from a much larger protein known as amyloid precursor protein (APP), the gene for which is located on chromosome 21. There appear to be a number of stages in the formation of senile plaques. Initially primitive plaques that lack any central amyloid are seen. These are followed by the more characteristic senile plaques, which have a central amyloid core surrounded by a shell of inflammation. In the final stage 'burnt-out' plaques are seen, which have just the core remaining with an outer shell of debris present as a result of the activity of scavenger cells within the brain. Further research is in progress to elucidate the sequence of action and whether the presence of plaques is the cause or the by-product of AD.

The senile plaques are found outside the brain cells, whereas neurofibrillary tangle formation is seen within the cell body. A protein known as tau protein is altered to form paired helical filaments which then clump together to form neurofibrillary tangles (*see* 2, colour plate section). As well as the presence of senile plaques and neurofibrillary tangles, other pathological changes that can be observed in AD includes neuronal loss, glial reaction, granulovacuolar degeneration, Hirano bodies in the hippocampus and white matter changes. Due to this progressive brain disease the structure of the brain cells is radically changed and the cells are unable to function normally. Eventually this leads to the death of brain cells and to the resulting clinical symptoms and signs of dementia.

Not surprisingly, as a result of the above neuropathological changes of AD taking place throughout the brain, and being quite marked in particular areas of the brain, the normal chemical balance of the brain is affected (Perl 2000; Wenk 2003). An imbalance in the neurotransmitters that are necessary to convey normal signalling and electrical charge from one brain cell to another leads to the clinical features of dementia. One of the main neurotransmitters to show a reduction in levels in AD is acetylcholine, and this has given rise to the *cholinergic hypothesis of AD*. There is a marked reduction in the activity of the enzyme involved in the synthesis of acetylcholine, namely choline acetyltransferase. Degeneration of cholinergic brain cells is associated with the density of senile plaques and the degree of dementia. Reduced levels of acetylcholine and decreased activity of the enzyme acetylcholinesterase (AChE, an enzyme that degrades acetylcholine) confirm the significant disruption of acetylcholine-related brain function. It would appear that as the acetylcholine-producing nerve cells die there is a reduction in the levels of this neurotransmitter, and a failure of transmission of the normal electrical impulses throughout the brain, leading to general brain dysfunction. A number of other brain neurotransmitters, such as noradrenaline and serotonin, have also been shown to be reduced in AD. The reduction in concentration of acetylcholine and these other neurotransmitters correlates with the increase in the number of senile plaques and neurofibrillary tangles.

Neuropathology of AD in DS

Probably the most well-established finding in the field of ID is that the brain of middle-aged and older adults with DS shows marked neuropathological changes of AD (*see* Table 2.1).

Prevalence of AD-like changes in DS

Ropper and Williams (1980), in a study of 24 people with DS aged 30 years or over, demonstrated neuropathological changes consisting of senile plaques and neurofibrillary tangles in the cerebral cortex. The severity of these changes increased with age. Only three individuals had dementia on clinical grounds. In a large study of 100 cases, the brains of institutionalised people with DS who died between 1950 and 1970 were studied retrospectively by Wisniewski *et al.* (1985).

Table 2.1 Studies of neuropathological changes of AD in DS

Authors	Number of subjects	Findings/comments
Malamud (1966)	347	Subjects over 40 years showed AD changes in all cases. In those under 40 years few cases showed AD change. AD changes increased with age
Burger and Vogel (1973)	13	AD changes in all but two cases
Ball and Nuttall (1980)	5	Changes of AD as compared to non-ID AD cases
Liss et al. (1980)	32	AD changes in all subjects over 30 years
Ropper and Williams (1980)	24	All subjects over 30 years showed AD changes
Sylvester (1984)	27	AD changes in 89% of subjects over 30 years, 95% over 40 years and 100% over 50 years
Wisniewski et al. (1985)	100	All subjects over 30 years and 7 under 30 years showed AD changes
Williams and Mattysse (1986)	23	All subjects over 30 years showed AD changes (except one case of possible DS)
Mann (1988)	18	Age-related AD changes
Motte and Williams (1989)	15	All cases except one over 40 years showed AD changes

A total of 51 patients were below the age of 30 years and 49 patients were above that age (age range 1–74 years). Brain weight, size and configuration appeared normal on examination for neonates and children up to the age of 4 years. The brain weight of patients over the age of 4 years was often 3% below the norm. A steady increase in AD changes was found with increasing age, particularly in patients over 30 years of age, with larger concentrations in the hippocampal cortex than in the prefrontal cortex.

Motte and Williams (1989), in a study of 15 patients with DS who were aged 25–59 years at the time of death, described the evolution of plaque morphology in the dentate gyrus. The earliest change (stage 1) was an extracellular accumulation of fibrillary material with histological characteristics of amyloid. This was followed by an 'exuberant neuritic reaction' with swollen processes that contained few or no paired helical filaments (stage 2). These two stages were predominantly seen below the age of 38 years. In stage 3 the neuritis showed signs of degeneration, with paired helical filaments surrounding a compact core of amyloid. The final stage (stage 4) consisted of a 'cloud of silver-positive debris'.

Mann (1988) reviewed previously published data along with their own data in order to determine the prevalence of neuropathological AD in DS. In 34 studies a total of 392 patients (age range 10–79 years) were studied, of whom 223 patients demonstrated AD changes. Of the 183 patients over 40 years of age, 180 individuals

Table 2.2 Age-specific prevalence of senile plaques and neurofibrillary tangles in DS

Age range (years)	Total number of patients	Number showing plaques and tangles	Percentage affected
0–9	37	0	0
10–19	79	6	7.6
20–29	58	9	15.5
30–39	35	28	80.0
Total < 39	209	43	20.6
40–49	50	49	98.0
50–59	87	85	97.7
60–69	43	43	100.0
70–79	3	3	100.0
Total > 40	183	180	98.4
Total	392	223	56.9

This table is based on the original that appeared as Table II, p. 103 in Mann DMA (1988) The pathological association between Down syndrome and Alzheimer disease. *Mech Ageing Dev.* **43**: 99–136.

(98.4%) had senile plaques and neurofibrillary tangles, whereas only 43 of of the 209 patients (20.6%) under the age of 40 years showed such changes (*see* Table 2.2).

The data in Table 2.2 suggest that there is an age-related increase in the incidence of senile plaques and neurofibrillary tangles, with a threshold point around the age of 30 years at which there is a dramatic and sudden change from a low incidence of AD changes (15.5% affected in the 20–29 years age group) to a high incidence (80% affected in the 30–39 years age group). The reason for this critical change remains unresolved, although future research specifically aimed at answering this question may prove to be of considerable clinical importance (Prasher 1994).

Distribution and density of lesions

At present it is generally accepted that the distribution pattern of lesions in adults with DS over the age of 40 years is similar to that in adults in the general population with AD (Crapper *et al.* 1975; Mann 1988; Cole *et al.* 1993). Senile plaque lesions can most frequently be found in the amygdala, hippocampus and associated areas of frontal and temporal cortex, with the visual, motor and sensory cortex being relatively spared. The distribution of neurofibrillary tangles follows essentially the same pattern, and they are also found in the limbic system, hypothalamus, periaqueductal region and pons.

The density of senile plaques and neurofibrillary tangles has previously been reported to be of similar magnitude in adults with DS to that in patients with AD in the general population (Ball and Nuttall 1980; Ropper and Williams 1980), or greater (Armstrong 1994; Hof *et al.* 1995). Subtle differences between the two populations may therefore be present (Alsop *et al.* 1986; Mann 1988).

Specificity of lesions

The high prevalence of senile plaques and neurofibrillary tangles in the brains of adults with DS over the age of 40 years appears to be specific to DS and not associated with the underlying ID *per se*. Malamud (1966) found no evidence of AD pathology in 588 non-DS patients with ID below the age of 40 years and in 31 (14%) of 225 patients over 40 years. To date, few cases of individuals with DS over the age of 50 years without histopathological evidence of AD have been reported. Usually these have been atypical karyotypes – for example, a 78-year-old woman with partial trisomy 21 (Prasher *et al.* 1998).

Vascular dementia

This is also known as multi-infarct dementia or arteriosclerotic dementia. In the general population it is the second commonest form of dementia after DAD. Approximately 20–30% of people who suffer from dementia have dementia associated with vascular disease. It occurs in younger individuals than is the case with DAD, and with a higher male:female ratio.

Vascular dementia usually involves narrowing of the arteries in the brain by arteriosclerosis leading to gradual impairment of brain function. Often patients with vascular dementia show other evidence of narrowing of the arteries elsewhere (e.g. presenting with heart disease, poor circulation in the legs, and hypertension). As a consequence of the narrowing of the arteries there is a constant reduction in blood flow, which can over time lead to damage to the brain nerve cells. Other forms of vascular dementia involve infarction in discrete areas of the brain where the brain cells are found to have degenerated. In this case the local blood supply has been cut off either due to a blockage, or to a rupture of the small blood vessels around that area. Sometimes this can be due to a blood clot (embolism) that has travelled some distance (from the heart or from the neck), leading to a blockage of the blood vessel in the brain and subsequent infarction. The area of infarction consists of dead brain cells which have thus lost their function. These changes can be visualised by brain neuroimaging techniques (computed tomography or positron emission tomography), in which areas of new pathology and old areas of damage can be seen.

The presentation and cause of vascular dementia are very different to those of DAD. Small infarcts and damage to the brain can occur over a number of years without any obvious clinical features. Decline can therefore be episodic rather than gradual as seen in DAD. There is therefore usually a stepwise decline. There may then be an acute episode, such as a stroke, or sudden onset of severe decline. Acute confusion can occur, which may resolve. In contrast to the situation in DAD, intellectual functioning in a person with multi-infarct dementia may remain quite stable or indeed improve over weeks or months, or over a number of years there may be deterioration. Certain areas of brain function, such as memory and speech, may be affected to a greater extent than personality or understanding (insight). The characteristic features of vascular dementia therefore include abrupt onset, stepwise deterioration, fluctuating course, episodes of confusion, relative preservation of personality, mood change, a history of hypertension or of strokes, evidence of vascular disease elsewhere, focal neurological signs, and focal neurological symptoms (e.g. gait abnormality, limb weakness).

Table 2.3 Hachinski Ischaemic Scale for Vascular Dementia*

Clinical feature	Number of points
Abrupt onset	2
Stepwise deterioration	1
Fluctuating course	2
Nocturnal confusion	1
Relative preservation of personality	1
Depression	1
Somatic complaints	1
Emotional incontinence	1
History of presence of hypertension	1
History of strokes	2
Evidence of atherosclerosis	1
Focal neurological symptoms	2
Focal neurological signs	2

*A score of 7 or more points is consistent with vascular dementia.

The risk factors for vascular dementia are similar to those for suffering a stroke, namely widespread atherosclerosis, hypertension, diabetes mellitus, smoking, hyperlipidaemia and heart arrhythmias or heart valve disease. Hachinski *et al.* (1975) published a scale to aid the clinical diagnosis of vascular dementia (*see* Table 2.3). Both vascular dementia and AD can occur together, a condition that is termed *mixed dementia*.

Lewy body dementia (LBD)

Lewy bodies are characteristic neuropathological changes seen in Parkinson's disease. They are small intracellular inclusion bodies which may be round or oval and have a distinct halo (*see* 5, colour plate section). However, they are also found in other forms of dementia in which AD or vascular changes are manifested. The clinical features are those of dementia, although individuals can present with parkinsonism, mental illness, fluctuating consciousness or falls. The cognitive decline that is seen in individuals with LBD is similar to that seen in DAD, but there are a number of specific differences:

- greater fluctuations in cognitive skills
- more marked day-to-day fluctuations in consciousness
- visual hallucinations (well formed and often persistent)
- depression
- parkinsonism (bradykinesia, limb rigidity, gait disturbances)
- frequent falls or faints
- sensitivity to neuroleptic medication.

The presence of Lewy bodies has been reported in the brains of adults with DS, but further research is required to investigate a possible association between these two conditions (Simard and van Reekum 2001). Raghavan *et al.* (1993) analysed the brains of 23 adults with DS (age range 31–74 years) for the presence of Lewy bodies. In two cases (aged 50 and 56 years) Lewy bodies were found in the substantia nigra. Bodhireddy *et al.* (1994) reported the case of a 54-year-old man with DS and dementia and marked parkinsonian signs that on neuropathological examination of the brain showed pathological changes of AD together with cortical Lewy bodies.

Frontotemporal dementia

Frontotemporal dementia is a common degenerative form of dementia. It encompasses several forms of dementia, in particular Pick's disease. There is marked degeneration of the frontal and temporal lobes. The clinical picture is similar to that in DAD, but there are several important differences:

- more marked early behavioural problems
- loss of awareness of the illness
- early marked personality change
- memory less affected.

Frontotemporal dementia, similar to vascular dementia, occurs in a younger population than DAD, and there is a more equal distribution between the sexes. Patients often first present with a history of behavioural or emotional change rather than memory loss. Symptoms may include loss of interest in usual day-to-day activities, disinhibition, a decline in self-hygiene, shoplifting, sexual impropriety, a change in eating behaviour, or emotional 'coldness' or indifference towards loved ones. The course and prognosis of frontotemporal dementia are quite similar to those for DAD.

Other types of dementia

Patients with *Parkinson's disease* are more susceptible to dementia. Parkinson's disease is principally a disorder of the deeper centres of the brain, where there is cell death and a reduction in levels of the neurotransmitter dopamine. A subsequent reduction in acetylcholine levels can occur, also leading to the presentation of dementia. *Dementia in Pick's disease* is a progressive dementia with onset reported for adults in the general population in middle age (50–60 years). There are initial changes in personality, followed by social deterioration. At a later stage, memory decline, impairment in language function and emotional change occur. *Dementia in Huntington's disease* usually follows the physical manifestation of Huntington's disease. In some cases, depression, paranoia or anxiety can be the earliest symptom. *Dementia due to human immunodeficiency virus disease* can present in a similar manner to DAD, but in a younger population. Seizures, tremor, ataxia, hypertonia and hyperreflexia are prominent features, and progression to death is rapid (sometimes occurring within weeks).

Causes of dementia

Among the general population, 10–30% of dementia cases have an identifiable cause which can be treatable and the dementia process can be reversed. Table 2.4 lists some of the common causes of dementia.

Table 2.4 Causes of dementia

Type of damage	Dementia type
Degeneration	Alzheimer's disease
	Dementia with Lewy bodies
	Frontotemporal dementia
	Parkinson's disease
	Huntington's chorea
Vascular disease with multiple infarcts	Multi-infarct dementia
	Binswanger's disease
	Cerebral amyloid angiopathy
Physical brain damage	Normal-pressure hydrocephalus
	Repeated head injury (e.g. due to boxing)
	Brain tumour
	Subdural haematoma
	Epilepsy
Toxic substances	Aluminium poisoning (particularly in dialysis)
	Wilson's disease
	Alcoholism
	Drug toxicity
	Medication-induced dementia
	Carbon monoxide poisoning
Endocrine disease	Diabetes mellitus
	Hypothyroidism
	Cushing's syndrome
	Systemic lupus erythematosus
	Hypercalcaemia
Infections	Bacterial meningitis
	Viral encephalitis
	Neurosyphilis
	Creutzfeldt–Jakob disease
Nutritional deficiency	Vitamin deficiency (vitamin B_{12}, folate, niacin deficiency)
Possible immune disease	Multiple sclerosis
	Polyarteritis nodosa

The degenerative and vascular causes of dementia have been reviewed above. In this section other, less common causes of dementia will be discussed.

Normal-pressure hydrocephalus

Hydrocephalus refers to the enlargement of the ventricular system within the brain. Normal-pressure hydrocephalus occurs when the flow of cerebral spinal fluid between the interior of the brain and the surface of the brain is partially or totally blocked following a head injury, meningitis or neurosurgery, or for an unknown reason. The blockage leads to eventual brain swelling and, due to the rigid skull, compression of the brain. As the blockage is not within the ventricular system, the intraventricular pressure remains normal or even low. Typical symptoms include intellectual deterioration, urinary frequency or incontinence, problems with walking and lack of coordination (Ojemann 1971). A lumbar puncture may be normal but an electroencephalogram recording should be abnormal, with random theta and delta activity. A computed tomography or magnetic resonance imaging scan will show marked ventricular dilatation with periventricular lucency around the anterior horns of the ventricles. A misdiagnosis of DAD can quite easily be made. This form of dementia may be reversible if a shunt is inserted to drain the fluid. This procedure involves inserting an indwelling catheter into the third ventricle and allowing the cerebrospinal fluid to drain via a one-way valve to the superior vena cava or peritoneal cavity. However, careful consideration is needed to determine which patients will benefit from this procedure, as complete recovery may only occur in one-third of individuals.

Tumour

Primary tumours (i.e. site of origin within brain) or secondary tumours (i.e. tumour has spread to brain from another part of the body) can cause dementia. The degree and prognosis will strongly depend on the nature of the tumour, its location, the severity of raised intracranial pressure and the general health of the individual concerned (Taphoorn and Klein 2004). The presentation will depend on the area of the brain involved, but generally the tumour may lead to gradual intellectual deterioration, personality or emotional change, and seizures with or without neurological signs. The clinical picture may be of typical dementia, but unusual symptoms (e.g. visual hallucinations), rapid deterioration or early onset, focal signs or features of raised intracranial pressure (e.g. vomiting, headaches, disturbed vision) should alert physicians to the need to perform a brain scan. Symptoms may be a direct result of the tumour, due to localised brain swelling or hydrocephalus, or alternatively even with large tumours no symptoms may be present. Misdiagnosis is not uncommon. Magnetic resonance imaging is the investigation of choice, as it can detect very small lesions that are not degraded by artefact and it can provide more detail with regard to the size of the tumour. The outcome will depend on the type, site and size of the tumour and whether it is amenable to neurosurgery.

Infections

General paralysis of the insane is due to chronic syphilis. This disorder is now rare, and it presents with a frontotemporal-type dementia (see above) and spinal cord disease. Dementia due to Creutzfeldt–Jakob disease (CJD) is a newly identified dementia that has been reported in older adults. A variant form of CJD occurs in young individuals, and is thought to be due to ingestion of meat contaminated with the transmissible prion. This disease has generated considerable public anxiety. Creutzfeldt–Jakob disease is a spongiform encephalopathy – a central nervous system disease caused by transmissible substances called prions. The typical presentation is in a young person with dementia, abnormal body movements (particularly jerking movements) and characteristic electroencephalogram changes. A biopsy and microscopic examination of brain tissue showing the spongiform neuropathological changes is necessary for definite confirmation of the disease. The prognosis is poor, with rapid deterioration over months rather than years.

Dementia due to human immunodeficiency virus is rare, but can occur in children as well as in adults. Dementia can be a direct result of the virus, or it may be due to a brain tumour or nervous system infections. The clinical picture involves forgetfulness, poor concentration, apathy and withdrawal, impaired walking, and delusions and hallucinations. Although it is usually part of the acquired immune deficiency syndrome (AIDS) complex, dementia can be the first manifestation of the syndrome.

Vitamin deficiency

Vitamin deficiencies as causes of dementia are uncommon, but may be more common in the ID population, who are vulnerable to poor nutrition. Neurological symptoms are common, and may present prior to any intellectual deterioration. Deficiencies in vitamin B_{12}, folic acid or niacin can lead to progressive dementia (Shulman 1967; Strachan and Henderson 1967). Vitamin B_{12} is necessary for the synthesis of myelin. When combined with intrinsic factor, which is produced by the parietal cells of the stomach, vitamin B_{12} is absorbed by the terminal ileum. Poor nutrition, a disorder of the ileum or a disorder of the stomach can lead to a reduction in vitamin B_{12} absorption. As well as causing dementia, vitamin B_{12} deficiency can lead to pernicious anaemia, combined degeneration of the spinal cord and psychosis. Folic acid deficiency can also cause depression and epilepsy. A raised mean cell volume (macrocytosis) may be found in patients with vitamin B_{12} or folic acid deficiency, but macrocytosis is also a common finding in healthy adults with DS and in older adults with DAD (Prasher et al. 2002a). All adults with ID who present with dementia should be screened for vitamin B_{12} and folic acid deficiency, as treatment can lead to an improvement in mental function (Henderson et al. 1966). Measurements of red cell folate levels are a better guide to long-term folic acid stores and are less affected by drugs.

Endocrine disorders

Endocrine disorders such as thyroid deficiency (hypothyroidism), parathyroid disease and diabetes mellitus may present as reversible forms of dementia. Historically, hypothyroidism was known to cause 'myxoedematous madness'. The disorder is more common in the elderly and can present with mental impairment, dulling of personality, apathy and slowing down, together with a number of physical symptoms suggestive of hypothyroidism, such as bradycardia, constipation, excess weight gain and dry coarse skin. Many of the physical symptoms may overlap with features of ID, thereby making the non-biochemical detection of hypothyroidism difficult. As thyroid deficiency is readily treatable, all individuals who present with dementia should be screened for a thyroid disorder.

Diabetes mellitus results from a deficiency of insulin, which causes hyperglycaemia and glycosuria. Poor diabetic control can lead to microvascular damage throughout the body, including the brain. The risk of DAD and vascular dementia is increased due to atherosclerotic brain infarctions, hypertension and cerebral anoxia. Diabetic management is complex, particularly in individuals with ID, and therefore considerable time and effort must be spent in educating the patient and their carers about the need for good control.

Endocrine deficiencies can be identified by laboratory tests. For hypothyroidism, low plasma levels of total and free thyroxine and raised levels of thyroid-stimulating hormone are characteristic. As up to one-third of adults with DS are known to have a thyroid dysfunction (Prasher 1999), all adults with ID who present with intellectual decline should be screened for a thyroid disorder. If psychological symptoms are treated early, the response to thyroxine replacement is good. However, replacement therapy should be undertaken gradually, as psychotic symptoms can occur with rapid treatment.

Hypoparathyroidism is an extremely rare condition but an important one that can present as progressive dementia (Robinson *et al.* 1954). The cause is commonly secondary to a thyroidectomy. Low serum calcium and high serum phosphate levels can be an indicator of the presence of hyperparathyroidism. Early treatment to correct the chemical imbalance can lead to marked improvement.

Medication

Many of the prescribed drugs in the field of mental health can impair cognition. These effects may be acute (e.g. confusion, drowsiness, ataxia and seizures) or more long-term (e.g. impairment of memory and concentration). Toxic effects may be idiosyncratic for any given individual, may result from interaction with a combination of drugs, or may be due to administration of excessive doses. Drugs that have been associated with the onset of dementia are listed in Box 2.2.

Box 2.2 Medications that have been associated with the onset of dementia

Anticonvulsants
   Sodium valproate
   Phenytoin
   Carbamazepine

Antipsychotics
   Chlorpromazine
   Thioridazine

Sedatives
   Barbiturates
   Benzodiazepines

Tricyclic antidepressants

Lithium

Older adults with ID are particularly susceptible to adverse effects. For any individual who presents with intellectual deterioration, prescribed medication should always be considered as a possible cause. Monitored controlled withdrawal of the medication can lead to improved intellectual functioning.

Chronic subdural haematoma

For individuals with ID, in whom falls and head injuries are more common than in the general population, a minor bump may lead to bleeding between the brain and the skull where a clot can form, which is termed a *chronic subdural haematoma*. Elderly people may have suffered a trivial injury several months earlier. The blood accumulates in the subdural space due to rupture of veins. Symptoms include fluctuating consciousness, headaches, ataxia and confusion, hemiparesis and visual defects. Late-onset seizures may be the first indication of an underlying chronic subdural haematoma. A misdiagnosis of a degenerative type of dementia is not uncommon. A skull X-ray may show a shift of the mid-line structures. A standard electroencephalogram recording may demonstrate a reduction in or loss of alpha rhythm over the affected site. Neuroimaging will indicate the site and severity of the haematoma (magnetic resonance imaging being superior to computed tomography). Early surgical evacuation can lead to full recovery, although treatment of long-standing chronic subdural haematoma will leave memory and intellectual impairment.

Other causes of dementia

There is evidence that repeated *head trauma* (e.g. as a result of recurrent falls) can lead to either parkinsonian-type dementia or DAD. The clinical presentation will depend on the degree and site of the head trauma. *Toxic damage* to the brain can lead to dementia. Poisons and metal toxicity (e.g. aluminium, lead) have also been reported as causes of dementia. Alcohol abuse can present with a wide range of intellectual disorders, including alcoholic dementia.

Summary

There is very little research in the field of ID investigating the prevalence and incidence of the different forms of dementia. Indeed in the scientific literature on ID there is a clear lack of clinical and neuropathological information on all but the commonest forms of dementia. The vast majority of research and clinical practice has focused on AD in adults with DS. There is now a need to investigate fully all individuals who present with intellectual decline, to enable as accurate a diagnosis as possible of the type of dementia.

Once a diagnosis of dementia has been made, it is important to detect the underlying cause of the dementia. In some cases a reversible cause (e.g. thyroid dysfunction, chronic subdural haematoma, brain tumour) will be found, treatment of which can have a significant effect in improving the quality of life of the individual concerned. A detailed assessment (*see* Chapter 4) of dementia is necessary to detect atypical symptoms or signs that can lead to the identification of the less common causes of dementia.

Chapter 3

Epidemiology of dementia

Introduction

Epidemiology is the investigation and study of disease in the context of a much larger population. Epidemiological research is particularly concerned with determining the frequency of the disease and its severity, and with identifying risk factors. Such research enables scientists to determine the importance of a given disease, allows services to be prioritised, and enables clinicians to determine causes with a view to finding appropriate treatments. Dementia, and in particular dementia in Alzheimer's disease (DAD), is a good example of a condition for which epidemiological research can help not only the population as a whole, but also affected individuals.

The quality of epidemiological research depends on a number of factors, in particular case definition and the sampling methods used. Case definition involves formulating a definition of an illness, and then identifying which individuals in a given population are diagnosed as having a particular disorder. In general medicine and surgery, a specific diagnostic laboratory test is often used to define 'caseness'. For example, a myocardial infarction will be defined by specific electrocardiogram changes on a Q-wave, ST elevation and T-wave inversion. When diagnostic tests are available, defining 'caseness' is not usually controversial. However, in the field of psychiatry, and particularly in the field of ID, defining when a person may have, say, DAD or schizophrenia can be contentious. In order to overcome such uncertainty, classification systems such as the *ICD-10* (World Health Organization 1992) and the *DSM-IV* (American Psychiatric Association 1994) have been developed.

Sampling methods involve the investigation of a subset of the total population, and it is assumed that findings for the subset can be extrapolated to the whole population. Classic epidemiological methods used in sampling include cross-sectional cohort and case–control studies. Sampling is vulnerable to sources of bias – for example, where undiagnosed cases are not included, or in rare cases (especially in tertiary centres) where there is over-inclusion of cases, giving much higher prevalence rates. Small sample size in the field of ID is an important source of bias.

Prevalence and incidence of dementia

At the start of the twenty-first century, in the USA approximately 10 million people have some form of dementia. The overall prevalence rate for the general population increases from approximately 5% at 65 years of age to over 50% at the age of 85 years. Dementia is uncommon below the age of 60 years. The number of individuals with dementia aged 85 years or over is expected to double within two

Table 3.1 Frequency of different types of dementia

Type of dementia	Frequency (%)
Alzheimer's disease	45–55
Mixed Alzheimer vascular diseases	15–25
Cerebral vascular diseases	5–15
Dementia with Lewy bodies	5–15
Reversible causes	3–7
Unknown causes	3–7

to three decades, leading to a huge economic burden. The prevalence of DAD in the general population is approximately 1.5% for the 65–69 years age group, increasing to around 20% for those over the age of 65 years.

A number of studies in the general population have investigated prevalence rates in individuals under the age of 65 years. Hofman *et al.* (1991) reviewed the prevalence of dementia in Europe reported in studies published between 1980 and 1990. They found specific prevalence rates of 0.1 for the 30–59 years age group, 1.0 for age 60–64 years, 1.4 for age 65–69 years, 4.1 for age 70–74 years, 5.7 for age 75–79 years, 13.0 for age 80–84 years, 21.6 for age 85–89 years and 33.4 for age 90–99 years. Thus for the general population DAD is very rare in young and middle-aged adults from the age of 30 years. However, there is a doubling in the rate of dementia approximately every 5 years after the age of 65 years.

The different types of dementia were discussed in Chapter 2. The relative frequency of the commonest forms of dementia in the general population is shown in Table 3.1.

A few studies have investigated the incidence of dementia in the general population in individuals below the age of 65 years. McGonigal *et al.* (1993) undertook a population study in Scotland using *ICD-9* (World Health Organization 1978) criteria. The incidence (expressed per 100 000 population at risk per year) of probable DAD was 1.44 for age 40–44 years, 27.6 for age 50–54 years and 37.8 for age 60–64 years. In a population-based study, Schoenberg *et al.* (1987) found the incidence of dementia to be 0.13% for the 60–69 years age group, 0.74% for the 70–79 years age group and 2.17% after the age of 80 years. Due to the relatively low rates for younger populations there are considerable difficulties in determining accurate incidence rates, and findings do vary considerably across studies. Certainly for the general population there is a steep increase in incidence with age, which is consistent with the increase in prevalence with age.

Age-associated cognitive decline or 'normal ageing' has recently been the subject of growing interest. Kral (1962) first introduced the term *benign senescent forgetfulness* to describe mild memory losses associated with age. Whether age-associated cognitive decline is part of the normal ageing process or early changes of DAD remains controversial. A Working Party of the International Psychogeriatric Association in collaboration with the World Health Organization proposed a set of criteria for diagnosing age-associated decline (Levy 1994). Features included the following:

- difficulties with memory and learning
- difficulties with attention and concentration

- readiness to confabulate
- visuo-spatial abnormalities.

An age-related decline in intellectual and adaptive skills that does not fulfil diagnostic criteria for DAD has been reported in adults with ID (Janicki and Jacobson 1986; Eyman and Widaman 1987, Prasher 1998). The classification of age-associated decline and its subsequent exclusion or inclusion as a form of DAD will undoubtedly affect both prevalence and incidence rates.

The increased survival of persons with ID, and in particular adults with DS, is the principal reason why DAD in the ID population is now not an uncommon occurrence (Zigman *et al.* 1997). Furthermore, with an increased survival rate for adults with dementia, the prevalence of dementia is now higher than previously. With improving medical and nursing care (in particular, antibiotics for chest infections, use of anti-dementia medication and improved carer support), people with dementia may continue to survive for on average a further 5 to 10 years after the initial onset of the disease. However, whether prolonging the life of a person whose quality of life continues to be poor can be regarded as 'progress' remains an area of significant moral and clinical debate.

Although the onset of dementia is age related, it can occur in individuals as early as the third decade of life. For individuals with DS, age-specific prevalence rates for DAD of 9.4% for the age range 40–49 years, 36.1% for age 50–59 years and 54.5% for age 60–69 years have been reported (Prasher 1995a). Several studies (*see* Figure 3.1) reported in the last 10 years have shown markedly higher age-specific rates for dementia in the DS population compared with the general population (Zigman *et al.* 1996; Holland *et al.* 1998; Tyrrell *et al.* 2001). The variation in reported rates in these studies is principally due to methodological differences.

Not only are adults with DS susceptible to developing DAD, but also it has been reported that the non-DS older population with ID are at risk of developing

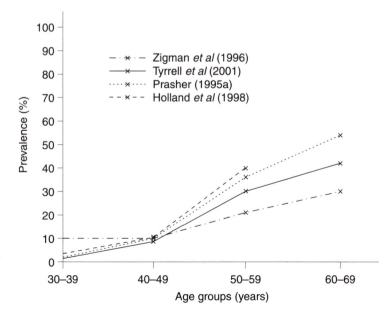

Figure 3.1 Recent studies demonstrating the prevalence of dementia in Down syndrome.

neuropathological changes of AD (Barcikowska *et al.* 1989; Popovitch *et al.* 1990). Baricikowska *et al.* (1989) examined post-mortem brain sections from 70 individuals with ID over the age of 65 years and found that 22 cases (31%) showed evidence of the presence of AD pathology. The rate was comparable to that seen in the general population at similar ages. There is limited information about the prevalence of clinical dementia in the non-DS elderly population with ID. Reported rates range from 6.1% to 21.6% (Patel *et al.* 1993; Cooper 1997a; Janicki and Dalton 2000) depending on the age cut-off for inclusion (50–65 years), the definition of dementia and whether the study was based on a survey or a case review. The most definitive study to have investigated the prevalence and incidence of dementia in non-DS individuals with ID was recently published by Zigman *et al.* (2004). The researchers conducted a longitudinal study in 126 adults over the age of 65 years. At intervals of 18 months, dementia status was assessed according to international guidelines (Aylward *et al.* 1997) using a battery of neuropsychological assessments, and data were collected over a 4.5-year period. The prevalence rates for dementia based on possible/definite dementia were 0.42 per 1000 for adults aged 65 years or over and 0.56 per 1000 for those aged over 75 years. The prevalence rates for DAD were 0.027 and 0.041, respectively. The consensus of opinion from the studies investigating the prevalence of dementia in the non-DS population is that the rate does not differ significantly from that for the general population.

Investigation of the incidence (new cases of a given disorder in an otherwise unaffected population) is notoriously difficult. Zigman *et al.* (2004) analysed the cumulative incidence rates for dementia and for DAD in their study. Only three new cases of possible/definite dementia were diagnosed during the study period, giving a cumulative incidence up to age 84 years of 0.08. The cumulative incidence of DAD based on two cases up to age 84 years was 0.06. These findings suggested that the incidence of dementia and DAD is not significantly higher (and could be lower) in older adults with non-DS ID compared with the rates for the general population (Bachman *et al.* 1993). Holland *et al.* (2000) reported the incidence of dementia in 68 adults with DS (mean age 42.3 years) to be 15 individuals aged 50 years or over but only three over 60 years of age. Subjects were assessed using a modified version of the Cambridge Examination for Mental Disorders of the Elderly (CAMDEX) (Roth *et al.* 1986) informant questionnaire, and repeat assessments were conducted 18 months after the initial ones. Over the 18-month period 13 individuals (24.5%) were given a diagnosis of dementia, of whom three fulfilled *ICD-10* criteria (World Health Organization 1992) for DAD.

Course and prognosis of dementia

The course and prognosis of dementia have implications not only for the person suffering from the disease, but also for services in terms of the cost of the illness and the need for further institutional care. For the general population a number of measures are available, such as the Clinical Dementia Rating Scale (Hughes *et al.* 1982) and the Global Deterioration Scale (Reisberg *et al.* 1988), which can assess the severity of dementia and be used to map the course of the deterioration over time.

The clinical course and the mortality rate for dementia are very much determined by the type of dementia that is present. For example, dementia associated with CJD may lead to death within a few weeks of the first symptom being detected. However, patients with DAD have been known to live for up to 20 years after diagnosis. Treves *et al.* (1986) investigated survival probabilities for DAD in individuals in the general population from the age of 65 years upward using life-table analysis. Approximately 30% of individuals had died from DAD by 5 years, and 85% by 10 years. The average life expectancy after diagnosis was 7–8 years.

Life expectancy for adults with DS who develop DAD appears to be not too dissimilar to that for the general population. It may possibly be shorter, or it may be that reported studies reflect the fact that the diagnosis of DAD in adults with ID is made later in the course of the disease, giving a false reduction in the time interval between onset and death. Wisniewski *et al.* (1985) examined seven patients neuropathologically and cognitively and found a mean duration of dementia of 5.6 years. Prasher and Krishnan (1993) reported that the mean age of onset of DAD in their review was 51.7 years, with a mean duration of 6 years. The mean age of onset for males was 53.6 years and that for females was 49.8 years (there was a statistically significant younger age of onset for females). Lai and Williams (1989) had earlier reported a mean age of onset of dementia of 54.2 years and an average duration of dementia of 4.6 years in 23 adults who died over an 8-year period. Discrepancies in reported life expectancy are primarily due to methodological differences. The majority of adults with DS who develop DAD can on average be expected to have a life expectancy of 4.0–7.5 years. There have been occasional reports in the scientific literature of adults surviving for up to 20 years.

Risk factors

A wide range of genetic and non-genetic risk factors for dementia have been investigated. With regard to genetic factors, the majority of research has focused on autosomal genes (see below). Numerous non-genetic factors have been investigated, but few have shown a consistent association. Environmental factors that have been studied include season of birth, smoking, thyroid disease, exposure to aluminium, level of education and head trauma (Forster *et al.* 1995; Bush and Beail 2004). A number of factors generally thought to be associated with DAD are discussed below. Genetic factors play a prominent role in the onset of dementia in individuals below the age of 65 years and in the DS population.

Age

It is well established that for the general population DAD is age related, the age-specific incidence of DAD doubling approximately every 5 years until the age of 85 years (Hofman *et al.* 1991). Other than in families with genetic mutations that predispose to early-onset DAD, DAD is extremely rare in adults below the age of 65 years in the general population (see discussion on epidemiology earlier in this chapter). The risk of DAD also increases with age in the ID population. With regard to the DS population, Prasher and Krishnan (1993) reviewed the scientific literature for 98 reports of dementia published between 1940 and 1990 and found that dementia was commonest in the fifth decade of life, but occasionally occurred in persons in their late thirties. The age distribution for DAD was

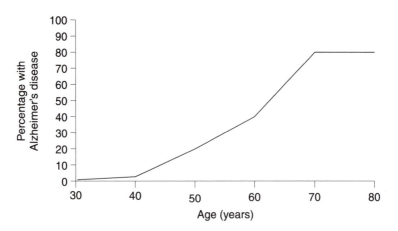

Figure 3.2 Survival curve for age of onset of dementia in people with Down syndrome.

skewed to an earlier onset by approximately 30 years for the DS population compared with the general population.

Zigman *et al.* (2004) confirmed that there was an increased risk of dementia with age in non-DS adults with ID, but this risk was significant after the age of 65 years. However, if it were not for the high mortality among the DS population after the age of 50 years, the increasing risk of DAD with age would reach 80% by the age of 70 years (*see* Figure 3.2).

It has not yet been fully determined why DAD is strongly related to increasing age. Is DAD a form of 'accelerated ageing' or is it a disease entity in its own right? Would all individuals develop DAD if they lived long enough? Clinical experience from both the general population and the ID population would suggest that many older adults could survive until old age without showing any evidence of DAD. For example, in a study by Prasher (1995a) of six adults with DS over the age of 70 years, only one person fulfilled the criteria for DAD. This would suggest that DAD (even in the high-risk DS population) is not inevitable.

Gender

Among the general population, prevalence studies suggest that women are affected by dementia to a greater extent than men. Specifically for DAD, a prevalence of 0.6% in males and 0.8% in females aged 60–65 years has been reported, increasing to 36% in males and 41% in females at the age of 95 years. However, this may reflect the increased life expectancy of women. Yet even when the increased female longevity is taken into account, there still appears to be a real female preponderance with regard to DAD. The influence of gender on the age of onset of DAD in the DS population has not been fully established. Some researchers (Prasher and Krishnan 1993; Raghavan *et al.* 1994; Lai *et al.* 1999) have suggested a greater risk and younger age of onset in females, while others have reported a greater risk and younger age of onset in males (Farrer *et al.* 1997; Schupf *et al.* 1998). Lai *et al.* (1999) investigated 100 adults with DS (aged 35–79 years), of whom 57 individuals had a diagnosis of dementia; women were 1.77 times more likely to develop dementia than men at any given point in time. This is in contrast to the findings of the study by Schupf *et al.* (1998), where males with DS were at higher risk for dementia than females. The cumulative incidence of dementia up to age 65 years was 0.79 in men with DS, compared with 0.28 for women.

Family history

For the general population there is an established strong familial risk for DAD (Heyman *et al.* 1984). Having a parent or sibling with DAD can lead to a two- to fourfold increased risk of DAD. The risk is even higher if more than one first-degree relative is affected, with a cumulative risk of 39–49% (Martin *et al.* 1988). Identical twins of an affected sibling are reported to be at highest risk (Jarvik *et al.* 1980). A few studies have reported that families of a relative with DAD are also at risk of having a relative with DS (Heston *et al.* 1981). Other researchers have found no such association (Amaducci *et al.* 1986; Huff *et al.* 1988). Conflicting findings have been reported with regard to a possible relationship between DAD and DS in first-degree relatives (Van Duijn *et al.* 1991; Schupf *et al.* 2001a). Schupf *et al.* (2001a) used survival methods to compare cumulative incidence and relative risk of DAD in the parents of 200 adults with DS and the parents of 252 adults with other forms of ID. The authors found that mothers who were 35 years of age or younger when their children with DS were born were four to five times as likely to develop DAD as control mothers. No association was found for mothers who were older than 35 years old when they gave birth to a child with DS. Sadovnick *et al.* (1994) investigated the incidence of birth of children with DS among offspring of women with DAD. The study assessed 578 liveborn offspring of 206 women with DAD. Data analysis showed that the frequency of DS live births, controlling for maternal age, to women who eventually developed DAD was not significantly different from that expected for the general population. Berr *et al.* (1989) investigated the prevalence of dementia in the families of 188 DS children and 185 controls. Rates of possible dementia were calculated for relatives over the age of 60 years (1336 individuals in the DS group and 1113 individuals in the control group). The rates of dementia were similar in the two groups (5.6% in the DS group and 6.2% in the control group). No excess of severe dementia was found in the families of children with DS. For individuals with DS there is limited information with regard to risk if family members are affected, but there is evidence that the risk is increased.

Vascular pathology

Not only can vascular pathologies (e.g. hypertension, diabetes, hyperlipidaemia) produce dementia in their own right or worsen AD pathology, but also it has been reported that vascular disease can be a risk factor for DAD. For example, hypertension has been reported to increase the risk of DAD (Skoog and Gustafson 2003). There is limited information in the literature regarding a possible association between DAD and vascular pathology in adults with ID. For adults with DS, Prasher and Blair (1996) found no association between low blood pressure and DAD, an association which had been reported for the general population.

Karyotypes

The majority of individuals with DS (95%) have non-disjunction trisomy 21. Virtually all reported cases of dementia have therefore been in these individuals.

However, the onset of dementia has been investigated in individuals with atypical DS karyotypes (translocations, mosaicism and partial trisomies). Several cases of DAD have been described in individuals with mosaic forms of DS (Whalley 1982; Sylvester 1986; Rowe *et al.* 1989), in an individual with a 21/22 translocation (Sylvester 1986), in a case with an unbalanced Robertsonian translocation 21/14 (Prasher 1993) and in another case involving a translocation 21/21 (Prasher 1996). There have been occasional interesting reports of elderly individuals with atypical DS who did not have DAD but lived to a relatively old age. Prasher *et al.* (1998) reported the case of a 78-year-old woman with DS with partial trisomy 21 [46,XX,rec(21)dup q, inv(21)(p12q22.1)] without evidence of DAD on neuropsychological, clinical or magnetic resonance imaging assessments. There was no evidence of DAD on neuropathological assessments. Quantitative Southern blot and fluorescence *in situ* hydridisation (FISH) analysis demonstrated that the gene sequence for the APP gene was present in only two copies. Chicoine and McGuire (1997) had earlier reported the case of a woman with DS who died at the age of 83 years, and who was free of dementia but showed 25% disomy for chromosome 21.

Head trauma

For the general population, conflicting results are available with regard to a possible association between head trauma and onset of DAD. Heyman *et al.* (1984) found an association, whereas Sulkava *et al.* (1985) found no such association. The EURODEM Risk Factors Research Group performed a group analysis of 11 different studies and found a pooled risk of 1.82 (95% confidence interval: 1.26–2.67) (Mortimer *et al.* 1991).

Pre-existing level of cognitive skills (severity of ID)

It has been postulated that a critical number of neurons must be present in the brain before DAD starts to develop. Once the number of neurons falls below this critical number a cascade process begins, resulting in DAD. Therefore, according to this hypothesis, the higher the intelligence level the greater the number of neurons in the brain prior to the onset of DAD, and the lower the risk of dementia. However, it remains controversial whether there is an association between onset of DAD and level of intelligence. Some studies in the general population have reported an increase in the risk of developing DAD in individuals who have had a low level of formal education (Sulkava *et al.* 1985; Fratiglioni *et al.* 1991). When other socio-economic factors were controlled for, the increased risk was reduced but still existed.

Reports of an association can be interpreted in several ways. First, a longer duration and higher level of education may induce greater life-long mental stimulation, which leads to physiological changes in the brain that reduce the risk of developing DAD. Secondly, there may be underlying brain dysfunction (possibly at birth) which leads to poor schooling and a lower level of education, and in later years to intellectual deterioration (dementia). Thirdly, a lower level of education may lead to susceptibility to other factors which cause dementia (e.g. nutritional deficiencies). Finally, the association between low level of education and increased risk of DAD may be an artefact (i.e. the poorer your intellectual skills the greater your chance of failing dementia neuropsychological tests).

Extrapolating the findings from the general population it would be expected that individuals with DS and severe ID would be at greater risk of developing DAD than those with moderate ID.

For the ID population, limited information is available regarding level of intelligence or ID and risk of dementia (Evenhuis 1990; Prasher 1997a; Temple *et al.* 2001). Prasher (1997a) reviewed case reports investigating clinical dementia in adults with DS that had been published between 1945 and 1995. For a total of 36 subjects, sufficient information was available about severity of ID, age of onset and duration of dementia. No statistically significant difference between age of onset, duration of dementia and severity of ID was found. For cases with moderate ID ($n = 19$) the mean age of onset of dementia was 46.9 years, and for those with severe ID ($n = 16$) the mean age of onset was 50.3 years. From the limited information available it would appear that, for adults with DS, education is not a major risk factor for DAD. Further prospective studies are needed.

Oestrogen deficiency

In older women with DAD, changes in gonadal hormones following the menopause have been postulated as a risk factor for the disease (Brenner *et al.* 1994; Tang *et al.* 1996). Oestrogen has been shown to promote the survival of cholinergic nerve cells (Toran-Allerand *et al.* 1992), although randomised controlled trials of oestrogen therapy have failed to show an improvement in cognitive skills in women with DAD (Henderson *et al.* 2000). The hormones of the hypothalamic–pituitary–gonadal axis, such as the gonadotropins (luteinising hormone and follicle-stimulating hormone), are involved in regulating reproductive function. Some researchers have proposed that it is the increase in gonadotropin levels rather than the decrease in oestrogen production following the menopause that results in an increased risk of DAD (Webber *et al.* 2004).

For women with DS, research studies have found a significant relationship between an earlier age of onset of the menopause and an increased risk of dementia (Cosgrave *et al.* 1999; Seltzer *et al.* 2001; Schupf *et al.* 2003). These findings support the hypothesis that a reduction in oestrogen levels may be a risk factor for the development of dementia.

Further ongoing research on the mouse model for DS suggests that oestrogen can alter amyloid precursor protein as well as dendritic and cholinergic markers, and that it can alleviate deficits (Granholm *et al.* 2003). At present it remains uncertain whether oestrogen deficiency is a significant risk factor for DAD. Indeed hormone replacement therapy has been reported to increase the risk of dementia (Pintiaux *et al.* 2003). Based on current evidence, hormone therapy is not indicated for the prevention of DAD in women with ID.

Genetics

For the general population a number of molecular studies have confirmed four (to date) specific genes that are associated with DAD, namely amyloid precursor protein (APP), the presenilins (PS1 and PS2) and apolipoprotein E (apoE). There is ongoing active research investigating the role of other possible genes. The APP, PS1 and PS2 genes cause DAD in an autosomal dominant pattern (95–100% penetrance), whereas apoE is a risk factor for DAD. However, in the general population less than 5% of the overall cases of DAD are due to APP or presenilin mutations. Apolipoprotein E status is a factor in all cases of DAD. For the ID population there is limited information on the role of genetics in the pathology of DAD (Schupf 2002).

Amyloid precursor protein (APP) gene

Since a mutation in the APP gene was first identified (Goate *et al.* 1991), considerable interest has focused on the association between the APP gene and AD (Clark and Goate 1993; Hendriks and van Broeckhoven 1996; Lendon *et al.* 1997; Levy-Lahad *et al.* 1998). The identification of an APP–AD-causing mutation gene came about because of the initial demonstration by researchers that the major protein of senile plaques found in AD was β-amyloid (a 39- to 43-amino-acid peptide) (Glenner and Wong 1984). Soon it was established that β-amyloid was derived by proteolytic processing from the β-amyloid precursor protein (Kang *et al.* 1987; Tanzi *et al.* 1987), and that the gene for APP was localised on chromosome 21 at 21q21.2 (Robakis *et al.* 1987; Tanzi *et al.* 1987). The commonest APP mutation is a valine/isoleucine substitution (Val717Ile). Studies of transgenic mice with APP mutations, in which there is increased deposition of β-amyloid and the presence of memory loss, further support an association between the APP gene and AD (Games *et al.* 1995).

Amyloid precursor protein is found throughout the body and its exact function is not known, but it has been postulated that it aids wound repair under normal physiological circumstances (Smith *et al.* 1990; Van Nostrand *et al.* 1990). Mutations in the APP gene can lead to disruption of this normal function by increasing cleavage of APP, which in turn leads to increased production of soluble amyloid, resulting in increased β-amyloid deposition (Lendon *et al.* 1997). However, the exact role of β-amyloid protein in the pathogenesis of AD continues to be controversial. Does β-amyloid protein accumulation cause neuronal degeneration and subsequent dementia, or is it a by-product of the pathogenic process? Evidence from studies of transgenic mice together with the finding that APP mutations are sufficient to cause AD in some cases would suggest the former.

Recent evidence has demonstrated the presence of at least two types of β-amyloid peptides, namely Aβ 1–40 and Aβ 1–42. Plasma levels of both types have been shown to be higher in adults with DS than in non-ID controls (Mehta *et al.* 1998; Schupf *et al.* 2001b; Head and Lott 2004). These peptides are formed from APP by sequential proteolytic cleavage by β- and γ-secretases. The β-secretase was recently identified as being the β-site APP cleaving enzyme 2 (BACE2), which is also located on the long arm of chromosome 21. Over-expression of BACE2 appears to be associated with AD neuropathology in adults with DS, and to be involved in amyloid β-protein production (Motonaga *et al.* 2002). The evidence would suggest that, as in adults in the general population with DAD, the diffuse plaques in adults with DS consist mainly of Aβ1–42, whereas Aβ1–40 is seen within the core plaques (Mann *et al.* 1995). Deposition of Aβ 1–42 has been reported to be a more important factor than deposition of Aβ 1–40 in the development of amyloidosis. It aggregates more readily than Aβ 1–40 and is deposited earlier in senile plaques (Iwatsubo *et al.* 1994).

The association between DS and the amyloid hypothesis of AD still requires further investigation (Head and Lott 2004; Margallo-Lana *et al.* 2004). As discussed in Chapter 2, during the latter half of the twentieth century it was established that virtually all individuals with DS who are over 40 years of age show the characteristic changes of AD on neuropathological examination (Mann 1988; Dalton and Wisniewski 1990). For the DS population it is postulated that over-expression of the APP gene leads to over-production of the amyloid precursor protein, resulting in excessive deposition of amyloid in the brain, with subsequent development of DAD. A number of immunological, neuro-pathological and clinical research studies support this hypothesis.

Prasher *et al.* (1998) published a detailed report of a single case that strongly supports this hypothesis. The report described a 78-year-old woman with DS who, on clinical examination, brain scanning and neuropathological assessment of her brain after death, showed no evidence of AD. Her karyotype demonstrated that she had a partial trisomy of the long arm of chromosome 21, which was cytogenetically confirmed to be 46,XX,rec(21)dup q, inv(21)(p12q22.1). Quant-itative Southern blot and FISH analysis demonstrated that the gene sequence for APP was present in only two copies. The patient was found to have an apoE 3 homozygous genotype.

Presenilin genes

The gene for PS1 is located on chromosome 14 and the gene for PS2 is located on chromosome 1. Over 100 families in the general population have been reported with DAD associated with over 40 PS1 mutations and 4 PS2 mutations (Cruts *et al.* 1998; Levy-Lahad *et al.* 1998). The age of onset of dementia in these families has been as young as 28 years, with virtually all individuals developing DAD by the age of 65 years. Deb *et al.* (1998) assessed whether PS1 polymorphic variations influenced age-specific rates of DAD in adults with DS over the age of 35 years. In a study of 26 adults with DS with DAD, 36 adults with DS without DAD and non-DS controls, no statistically significant difference was observed in any of the inter-group comparisons. Tyrrell *et al.* (1999) also found no significant association between PS1 polymorphisms and DAD in a study of 231 adults with DS over the age of 35 years.

Apolipoprotein E

Apolipoproteins are important proteins, synthesised by the liver, that aid the transfer of cholesterol and other lipids from one cell to another. Apolipoprotein E is found in the brain and is an essential lipoprotein for normal lipid homeostasis during myelination and cell membrane repair (Lendon *et al.* 1997). It is the only lipoprotein that is synthesised in the brain (by astrocytes). Apolipoprotein E is produced by a single gene located on chromosome 19 (19q13.2). This gene has three different alleles (ε2, ε3 and ε4) which are inherited from each parent, leading to the formation of three forms of apoE (apoE2, apoE3 and apoE4) with six genotypes (E2/E2, E2/E3, E2/E4, E3/E3, E3/E4 and E4/E4). The distribution of alleles found in the Caucasian population has been reported to be of the order of 7–10% for ε2, 70–80% for ε3 and 10–15% for ε4 (Van Duijn *et al.* 1995).

There is now a consensus that possession of the apoE ε4 allele predisposes the general population to DAD, whereas the presence of apoE ε2 may protect the general population from development of the condition (*see* Table 3.2). The risk of DAD associated with apoE genotype is dose dependent, one copy of apoE ε4 increasing the risk of DAD by 2.2–4.4 and two copies conveying an increased risk of 5.1–17.9 (Corder *et al.* 1993; Tsai *et al.* 1994). The mean age of onset of DAD for

Table 3.2 Studies investigating the association between apolipoprotein E status and DAD in the general population

Study	Number of DAD subjects	Mean age (years)	Findings
Corder *et al.* (1993)	97	70.9	ApoE $\varepsilon4$ gene dose is risk factor for late-onset DAD
Liddell *et al.* (1994)	86	73.5	Increased prevalence of $\varepsilon4$ allele in patients with DAD. Odds ratio in homozygotes for $\varepsilon4$ allele was 11.24
Talbot *et al.* (1994)	93	75.0	Increased prevalence of $\varepsilon4$ allele in DAD subjects. Decrease in $\varepsilon2$ allele frequency. ApoE $\varepsilon2$ has protective effect against DAD
Tsai *et al.* (1994)	77	80.5	ApoE $\varepsilon4$ allele frequency higher in DAD subjects. Median age at onset decreased as number of apoE $\varepsilon4$ alleles increased from 0 to 1 to 2
Van Duijn *et al.* (1995)	175	63.0	ApoE $\varepsilon2$ is associated with increased risk for early-onset DAD and reduced survival
Kukull *et al.* (1996)	234	80.2	Heterozygous $\varepsilon4$ had odds ratio of 3.1 for DAD compared with no $\varepsilon4$. Homozygous $\varepsilon4$ subjects had odds ratio of 34.3
Duara *et al.* (1996)	197	75.0	No significant differences in ApoE $\varepsilon4$ frequency in different ethnic groups. ApoE $\varepsilon4$ associated with family history of DAD but not gender or educational status
Gomez-Isla *et al.* (1996)	359	77.8	ApoE $\varepsilon4$ associated with earlier onset of DAD but not rate of progression
Murphy *et al.* (1997)	86	65.3	No association between ApoE $\varepsilon4$ and rate of cognitive decline

individuals inheriting the apoE 4/4 genotype is less than 70 years, whereas the mean age of onset for individuals inheriting the apoE 2/3 genotype is over 90 years (Strittmatter and Roses 1996). Each $\varepsilon4$ allele will lower the age of onset of DAD by up to 9 years (Strittmatter *et al.* 1993). Although some researchers suggest that the presence of an apoE $\varepsilon4$ allele accelerates the progression of DAD (Kanai *et al.* 1999), the majority have found that the apoE4 genotype does not affect the severity or duration of the disease process (Corder *et al.* 1995; Growdon *et al.* 1996; Slooter *et al.* 1999). However, it must be borne in mind that $\varepsilon4$ is neither necessary nor sufficient for the onset of DAD. Many individuals develop DAD but do not have an $\varepsilon4$ allele, and similarly individuals with an $\varepsilon4$ allele have been known to survive to advanced years without the onset of DAD. This would suggest that different factors influence the onset of DAD compared to those that determine its progression.

The role of apoE genotyping in the diagnosis of DAD remains controversial. The sensitivity in post-mortem studies with small sample sizes has been reported to be 46–78% (Saunders *et al.* 1996). Mayeux *et al.* (1998) reported a study reviewing clinical and pathological diagnoses of dementia with apoE genotype from 26 centres in the USA. The sensitivity and specificity for 1833 patients with a clinical diagnosis of DAD and for 1770 patients with a pathological diagnosis of AD were determined. In total, 62% of patients with a clinical diagnosis had at least one apoE ε4 allele, as did 65% of those with a pathological diagnosis. The sensitivity of the apoE ε4 allele for a clinical diagnosis of DAD was 93%, and its sensitivity for a pathological diagnosis of AD was 65%. The specificity was 55% and 68%, respectively. The authors concluded that as a diagnostic test for DAD, apoE genotyping did not have sufficient sensitivity and specificity. However, when used in combination with clinical criteria the researchers found that it could significantly improve the accuracy of the diagnosis.

Following the establishment of a strong association between the apoE genotype and DAD in the general population, several researchers have investigated an association in the DS population (*see* Table 3.3). Compared with studies in the general population, studies of adults with DS have usually involved small numbers of subjects, often with few cases of DAD, poor diagnostic criteria for clinical dementia and inappropriate selection of control groups. From the available data, the role of the apoE genotype in the development of DAD in adults with DS remains uncertain and less dramatic than in the general population.

Some studies have reported no significant association between the presence of the apoE ε4 allele and DAD in the DS population (Van Gool 1995; Wisniewski *et al.* 1995; Lambert *et al.* 1996; Prasher *et al.* 1997; Tyrrell *et al.* 1998), while others have reported a possible association (Royston *et al.* 1994; Martins *et al.* 1995; Schupf *et al.* 1996; Sekijima *et al.* 1998; Deb *et al.* 2000).

Also still controversial are the possible protective effects of the apoE ε2 allele on onset of DAD in adults with DS. Some reports suggest that there may be a protective effect (Hardy *et al.* 1994; Royston *et al.* 1994; Schupf *et al.* 1996; Tyrrell *et al.* 1998), but due to the low frequency of the ε2 allele in this population the power calculation has often been too small to allow appropriate data analysis. For similar reasons it remains difficult to demonstrate unequivocally whether the presence of an apoE ε4 allele lowers the age of onset of DAD in adults with DS, as has been reported in some studies (Schupf *et al.* 1996; Tyrrell *et al.* 1998). Van Gool *et al.* (1995) in their limited study found no association between apoE status and duration of DAD.

However, further studies of larger samples of DS cases that fulfil recognised diagnostic criteria for DAD are required. Studies of definite cases of DAD may clarify the previous conflicting results of studies investigating the role of apoE status. The effects of apoE status on the progression of DAD can best be investigated by prospective longitudinal studies, ideally following individuals up to the point of death.

Summary

Dementia in Alzheimer's disease is of major concern both to the general population services and to services for people with ID. The disorder is particularly

Table 3.3 Reports of apoE allele frequency versus clinical dementia in adults with DS

Study	DS subjects with clinical dementia Allele frequency (%)				DS subjects without clinical dementia Allele frequency (%)			
	Total	ε2	ε3	ε4	Total	ε2	ε3	ε4
Royston et al. (1994)	34	1(3%)	25(74%)	8(23%)	10	5(50%)	5(50%)	0(0%)
Wisniewski et al. (1995)	30	2(7%)	28(93%)	0(0%)	32	3(9%)	28(88%)	1(3%)
Van Gool et al. (1995)	52	3(6%)	42(81%)	7(13%)	52	6(11%)	41(79%)	5(10%)
Martins et al. (1995)	12	1(8%)	7(59%)	4(33%)	34	5(15%)	28(82%)	1(3%)
Lambert et al. (1996)	16	1(6%)	13(81%)	2(13%)	54	7(13%)	40(74%)	7(13%)
Schupf et al. (1996)	26	0(0%)	18(69%)	8(31%)	138	12(9%)	109(79%)	17(12%)
Prasher et al. (1997)	17	4(12%)	28(82%)	2(6%)	83	11(7%)	135(81%)	20(12%)
Sekijima et al. (1998)	32	2(6%)	24(75%)	6(19%)	174	4(2%)	158(91%)	12(7%)
Tyrrell et al. (1998)	31	0(0%)	51(82%)	11(18%)	60	10(8%)	97(81%)	13(11%)
Lai et al. (1999)	57	5(4%)	89(78%)	20(18%)	43	11(13%)	64(74%)	11(13%)
Rubinsztein et al. (1999)	20	1(5%)	32(80%)	7(15%)	25	3(6%)	40(80%)	7(14%)
Deb et al. (2000)	24	0(0%)	40(83%)	8(17%)	33	3(5%)	57(86%)	6(9%)

associated with DS and affects the majority by the age of 55 years. The number of older adults with DS in the community may be small but is growing. All of these individuals have a very high risk of DAD compared with their non-ID counterparts. Further research is required to fully determine the incidence, outcome factors and prognostic indicators for adults with ID who develop dementia. There is still a lack of information on dementia in non-DS individuals with ID, and on the epidemiology of forms of dementia other than DAD. Considerable research is needed to study population-based disease in the ID population. Few large-scale community-based studies investigating a wide range of risk factors for DAD in the ID population have been undertaken. Some of the risk factors for DAD appear to be equally applicable to both populations (e.g. age), while other factors have a greater effect in the general population (e.g. apoE genotype, family history of DAD).

Chapter 4

Clinical presentation of dementia

Introduction

Dementia is characterised by the development of a wide range of cognitive and non-cognitive features which are influenced by age, gender, level of underlying intelligence, premorbid disorders, medication and the surrounding environment. Therefore, although there are 'typical' features of dementia, it must be borne in mind that these features are significantly affected by the above factors, and presentation may vary markedly between individuals. In adults with intellectual disabilities (ID), early symptoms and signs of dementia may be difficult to detect. This is because of the underlying intellectual impairment, as a result of which the early detection of characteristic features of dementia, such as short-term memory loss and impairment of concentration and attention, may be difficult to elicit. Furthermore, the underlying cause of the dementia will lead to different clusters of symptoms and signs being associated with different forms of dementia. For adults with ID, dementia is particularly associated with Down syndrome (DS), and the principal underlying cause of dementia is that of Alzheimer's disease (DAD). Very few conditions can give rise to such marked changes as those seen in progressive DAD (*see* 6, 7, 8 and 9 colour plate section). In Chapter 2 the characteristic features of the different types of dementia were discussed. This chapter will primarily focus on dementia in Alzheimer's disease.

Overall presentation

The definition of dementia is discussed in Chapter 2. To summarise, dementia is a disease of the brain that is usually progressive, leading to impairments in cognition, emotion and behaviour, with marked deterioration in social function. The common features of DAD are listed in Box 4.1.

Box 4.1 Signs and symptoms of dementia

Forgetfulness
Disorientation
Apraxia
Aphasia
Agnosia
Impaired recognition
Impaired judgement
Changes in mood
Disturbed behaviour

Delusions
Hallucinations
Disturbed sleep
Seizures
Incontinence
Wandering

Dalton and Crapper-McLachlan (1986) reviewed 35 case reports of people with DS for whom a clinical description had been given in relation to the development of dementia. In total, 33 cases showed clear post-mortem evidence of AD, of whom five showed no evidence of dementia while alive. The most frequently occurring symptom/sign was the presence of epilepsy (88% of subjects), followed by focal neurological signs (46%) and personality change (46%). Other symptoms and signs were (in order of frequency) incontinence, apathy, inactivity, loss of conversation, electroencephalogram changes, loss of self-help skills, tremor, myoclonus, visual or auditory effects, walking impairment, stubbornness, uncooperative behaviour, depression, memory loss, posture of flexion, increased muscle tone, disorientation and hallucinations or delusions. However, there were many instances of unreported signs, which calls into question the accuracy of the above list.

Lai and Williams (1989) studied 96 individuals with DS over the age of 35 years. Treatable causes of dementia (hypothyroidism, neurosyphilis, vitamin B_{12} deficiency, brain tumour) were excluded. Three phases of clinical deterioration were recognised. In the initial phase, memory impairment, temporal disorientation and reduced verbal output were evident in the higher-functioning individuals with DS. For the more disabled patients, the first indications of dementia were apathy, inattention and reduced social interactions. In the second phase, loss of self-help skills such as dressing, toileting and use of eating utensils was seen. The gait was often slowed and shuffling. In the final phase the patients were non-ambulatory and bed-ridden, often assuming flexed postures. Sphincter incontinence was present and pathological reflexes such as sucking, palmar grasp and glabellar reflexes were prevalent. Parkinsonism developed in 20% of cases. Seizures occurred in 41 (84%) of the 49 demented patients, but were present in all 23 individuals who died. Four patients had a pre-existing seizure disorder, 23 cases had the onset within two years of mental decline, and in 14 cases seizures developed more than three years after the dementia began. Most of the seizures were of a generalised and tonic–clonic type, and several patients had partial complex seizures, but all were easily controlled with anticonvulsants. Seven patients also developed myoclonus. Ten patients (20%) in the demented group had the flexed posture, bradykinesia, masked face and cogwheel rigidity of parkinsonism, and four patients had a coarse resting tremor.

These findings were confirmed in a prospective longitudinal study by Evenhuis (1990). Of the 17 patients who were studied (age range 45–63 years; 7 men and 10 women), dementia was diagnosed clinically in 15 patients, who showed deterioration in daily living skills and fulfilled modified DSM-III-R criteria (American Psychiatric Association 1987) for dementia. Autopsy confirmation was obtained in eight cases. Early symptoms of dementia included apathy, social

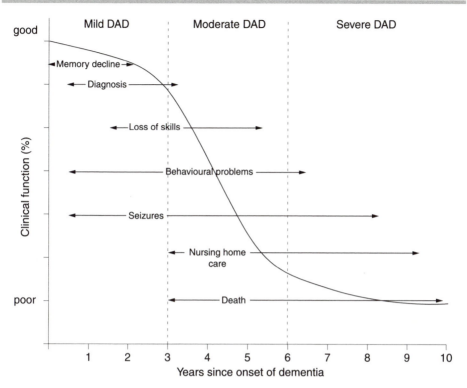

Figure 4.1 Course of dementia.

withdrawal and loss of self-help skills. Severely disabled patients presented with gait deterioration, myoclonus and epileptic seizures as early signs. Deterioration of speech occurred in a high proportion of cases.

Cosgrave *et al.* (2000) undertook a 5-year follow-up study of 80 female subjects to determine the symptoms and patterns of deterioration over time. During the study period the number of subjects with a diagnosis of DAD increased from 7 to 35. Trigger symptoms of dementia included memory loss, spatial disorientation, epilepsy, urinary incontinence, gait abnormality, apathy and increasing impairment of activities of daily living.

The duration and prognosis of DAD in adults with DS were discussed in Chapter 2. Dementia in Alzheimer's disease is a debilitating disease that leads to marked clinical change (*see* Figure 4.1). The terminal stage of DAD consists of severe intellectual deterioration, marked personality and mood changes, loss of sphincter control, seizure activity, immobility with hypertonia, and complete loss of self-care skills (Prasher 1995b).

Non-cognitive features

The non-cognitive psychopathology of DAD has been well established in the general population as being an integral part of the dementing process. In the field of ID, cognitive and adaptive behavioural change has often taken prominence. However, carers themselves frequently report that it is the non-cognitive and behavioural features which are of particular concern. Moss and Patel (1995) reported on psychiatric psychopathology using the Psychiatric Assessments Schedule for Adults with Development Disability (PAS-ADD) (Moss *et al.* 1993), a semi-structured psychiatric interview questionnaire. A total of 18 individuals from a sample of 99 subjects were judged to have probable dementia, of whom 12 patients had confirmed dementia. The authors found that individuals with dementia were more likely to score positively on loss of interest, sleep difficulty, irritability, slowness, and poverty of speech. However, the PAS-ADD questionnaire did not include items for assessing psychotic features.

Memory impairment

Deterioration in short-term memory is often the principal feature required to make a diagnosis of DAD. For the adults in the general population it is usually the earliest presenting symptom. People with DAD have difficulties in learning new material and retaining new information, and they tend to forget previous information that they would normally have remembered, particularly recent information. Individuals may lose items, forget to follow commands or instructions or become unfamiliar with known places. As the dementing process progresses, the short-term memory loss increases in severity to the point where a person may no longer recognise relatives or long-standing carers, and may forget their own birthday and sometimes even their own name.

It is not unusual for a person from the general population who develops DAD to highlight difficulties in their own memory. However, relatively high levels of intellectual skill and insight are required by older adults with ID who develop DAD for this to occur. Often it is carers with whom they have regular contact (paid carers or family members) who first become aware that there is a presenting problem, and who may seek help for this. An interview with carers is usually necessary to elicit information and examples that suggest memory deterioration. More formal neuropsychological testing can be undertaken in order to assess the registration, retention, recall and recognition of information which may demonstrate the cognitive deterioration associated with DAD (*see* Chapter 5 for details of neuropsychological testing).

The ability to learn new information can be assessed by asking the individual to remember a new list of words or a list of pictures. They can be requested to repeat given words (registration), then be asked to recall the information after a few minutes (retention, recall), and later on asked to recognise the words from a much longer list (recognition). Prompts may be required to enable the person to recall items. Long-term (remote) memory is not usually impaired at an early stage of DAD, and it is not uncommon for carers themselves to state how amazed they are that the person cannot remember what they had for breakfast, but can remember the names and addresses of places where they used to live when they were young adults.

When assessing and becoming aware of problems with cognition, it is clinically important to assess the impact of the deficits on the individual's social and personal lifestyle. The impact is usually less than that for the general population, as older people with ID are often not independent, many of their activities being either performed under supervision or done for them (e.g. having their meals prepared for them, being transported to their day activities, being supervised with regard to bathing and hygiene). Furthermore, in the past older people with ID often spent most of their lives in institutions and therefore never had the opportunity to develop independent skills. Therefore older adults living semi-independently in the community are more likely to give cause for concern and are more likely be diagnosed with DAD early on.

Historically, a number of studies have documented memory deterioration in older adults with DS. Dalton and Crapper-McLachlan (1984) devised a delayed match-to-sample memory test in their study, which was conducted over an 8-year period to investigate dementia in adults with DS. The average age of onset of memory impairment was 49.1 years (range 41–60 years). The authors concluded that the delayed match-to-sample performances could be used as valid behavioural markers to detect dementia. Brugge *et al.* (1994) investigated cognitive impairment in adults aged 20 to 51 years with DS along with controls. A number of neuropsychological assessments were undertaken, but the authors found that the short delayed saving score from the Californian Verbal Learning Test (a test of verbal memory) was a sensitive cognitive marker for early DAD. Devenny and colleagues (Devenny *et al.* 2000; Krinsky-McHale *et al.* 2002) investigated the sequence of cognitive decline in dementia in adults with DS. They found that adults with early-state dementia showed a decline on the object assembly, picture completion, arithmetic and comprehension sub-tests of the Wechsler Intelligence Scale for Children (Revised) (Wechsler 1974), while adults with middle-stage dementia showed a decline in the same sub-tests together with declines in information, vocabulary and digit-span sub-tests. Furthermore, Devenny *et al.* (2000) went on to investigate changes in verbal explicit memory using the selective reminding test in adults with DS, some of whom had an *ICD-10* (World Health Organization 1992) diagnosis of DAD. The authors found that the modified version of the Selective Reminding Test (Buschke 1973) could detect memory changes.

Devenny *et al.* (2002) evaluated memory decline with an adaptation of the Cued Recall Test (Buschke 1984) in 19 adults with DS who were at an early stage of DAD, and their performance was compared with that of controls. Eight of the DS adults with DAD performed relatively poorly on the Cued Recall Test compared with their healthy peers at a baseline when functional decline was not suspected. This finding suggested that memory decline could occur several years prior to the identification of DAD.

Deterioration in language function

Deterioration of language (aphasia) may present in individuals with DAD as difficulty in verbalising the names of objects or individuals or in being able to answer simple questions (Emery 2000). Speech in adults with DAD is slowed down, the flow of speech may be disrupted, and individuals may be seen deliberately trying to recall the answer to questions and trying to name things. The comprehension of spoken language can also be affected, and individuals may not carry out simple commands. As DAD becomes severe, the affected person may become mute, or they may present with echoing speech they have heard (echolalia), or repeating sounds and words (palialia). As with memory, carers themselves may give a history of such problems. Simple questions can be asked to elicit deficits. For example, individuals can be asked to name objects during the interview (e.g. watch, pen, tie). The ability to understand commands can be assessed by asking the person to put their hand on their head or to close their eyes.

Kledaras *et al.* (1989) monitored picture naming longitudinally in a 59-year-old man with DS with diagnosed dementia. During the test he was shown a series of 40 pictures, and his task was to say their names. The test was repeated periodically over the course of approximately 2 years. Initially 100% correct scores were achieved, and accuracy was maintained until the tenth month. From this point onward his scores gradually declined until he scored less than 30% correct on the final test.

Personality change

Personality change occurs in all adults with DAD. It may precede cognitive decline and occur several years before a formal diagnosis of DAD is made. The affected individual may become more irritable and hostile than previously. Aggression and anger may predominate and be associated with difficult behaviour. Some patients can become more placid and amenable when previously they were more awkward and stubborn. Anxiety is common and may be a reaction to a change in routine, or to a change in circumstances or environment such that the person is placed in a situation with which they are unfamiliar. Anxiety would have an add-on effect to impairment of functional ability and would further impair adaptive behaviour. Associated with the emotional changes there may be what is termed 'emotional lability' – that is, frequent and unpredictable changes in emotion (e.g. a person becoming tearful, happy or irritable) with little apparent reason.

Behavioural difficulties

Behavioural symptoms are a common feature of dementia in the general population. Cooper (1997b) investigated maladaptive behaviour in older adults with ID, and compared 29 individuals with dementia with 99 individuals without dementia. Behaviours that were significantly more common in the dementia group included lack of energy, lack of sense of danger, sleep disturbance, agitation, incontinence, excessive lack of cooperation, mealtime/feeding problems, irritability and aggression. Cooper and Prasher (1998) compared non-cognitive symptoms in DS individuals with dementia versus non-DS ID individuals with dementia. The DS group had a higher prevalence of low mood, restlessness, excessive overactivity, disturbed sleep, excessive lack of cooperation, and auditory hallucinations. However, aggression occurred more commonly in the non-DS demented group.

Prasher and Filer (1995) investigated behavioural change in adults with DS who were matched with non-demented DS controls. Changes in mood, communication difficulties, gait deterioration, loss of self-care skills, sleep disturbance, daytime wandering and urinary incontinence were particularly associated with DS individuals with DAD. Problems that caused greatest concern for carers were restlessness, loss of communication skills, urinary incontinence and wandering.

Non-cognitive features of dementia present a challenge to carers, particularly elderly carers. Persistent aggression, disturbed sleep and excessive lack of cooperation can lead to considerable distress and burden for family carers.

Behavioural features appear to be associated with dementia in all individuals with ID, irrespective of the cause of the latter, although people with DS may have a particular profile of behavioural problems. There is a need for health and social services to provide appropriate treatment in order to reduce symptoms, whether by means of pharmacotherapy, behavioural therapy or social change.

Agitation and aggression

In this chapter a broad definition of agitation and aggression is used. This covers verbal and physical behaviours, along with a number of inappropriate behaviours (*see* Box 4.2). Agitation and aggression occur in the majority of adults in the general population with DAD, and also in a significant proportion of adults with dementia in the ID population. There is a strong overlap between agitation and aggression, and the two issues will be discussed together. Agitation and/or aggression is more likely to occur in the early or middle stages of DAD, particularly when the individual is more active and mobile. During the latter stage of the dementing process when the individual is more immobile, agitation and behavioural aggression are less disruptive. It is not unusual for carers to be more concerned about aggressive behaviour in an ID adult with dementia than about the degree of memory loss or other cognitive decline.

Box 4.2 Types of agitation and aggression

Screaming
Shouting
Repeated requests
Hitting
Grabbing
Pushing
Pinching
Kicking
Throwing objects
Biting
Smearing faeces
Sexual exposure

Depressive symptoms

It is reported that in the general population depressive symptoms can be an early presentation of DAD or, as is argued by some researchers, can predispose individuals to DAD (Burns 1991; Teri and Wagner 1992). It remains uncertain whether the onset of depression is a psychological response to impending memory and cognitive loss or a manifestation of the underlying AD process (Pearlson *et al.* 1990). Burt *et al.* (1992) reviewed depressive psychopathology and the onset of dementia in adults with ID, and found that a number of symptoms associated with dementia were also associated with depression (*see* Box 4.3).

Box 4.3 Depressive symptoms seen in dementia

Inactivity
Loss of self-help skills
Depression
Urinary incontinence
Irritability
Slowing
Uncooperative or unmanageable behaviours
Loss of housekeeping skills
Greater dependency
Loss of way and recognition of surroundings
Weight loss
Emotional deterioration
Destructiveness
Hallucinations – delusions
Sleep difficulties

The authors reported a strong overlap between the clinical features of depression and dementia in adults with DS, and stated that this association was greater than for the general population. Prasher (1995a) confirmed the findings of Burt *et al.* (1992) in a study of 201 adults with DS, of whom 27 individuals had an *ICD-10* (World Health Organization 1992) diagnosis of DAD. The depressive symptoms of mental deterioration, disturbed sleep pattern, weight loss, motor retardation, reduced speech output, reduced appetite and depressed mood were all significantly more common in demented than in non-demented individuals. Certainly the depressive symptoms seen in adults with ID with dementia can fulfil the clinical criteria for a depressive episode (Prasher and Hall 1996; Sung *et al.* 1997).

The management of a depressive illness in a person with ID who has dementia is not too dissimilar to that for a younger adult with ID and without dementia. A full detailed history should be taken together with a detailed mental state and physical examination, and additional information from standard assessment. A trial of antidepressant medication may lead to intellectual improvement and further clarify the diagnosis. Psychotherapy and behavioural therapy may also be necessary, along with support for carers and continued ongoing support in the community. Advice on how to maintain a good appetite and healthy body weight can be given by the speech and language therapist and/or occupational therapist.

Perceptual changes (delusions and hallucinations)

In his original report of a woman with dementia, Alzheimer (1907) described the psychotic features of delusions and hallucinations. Subsequent research studies have suggested that up to 50% of adults in the general population with DAD can present with delusions (Cummings *et al.* 1987), with up to 76% presenting with either auditory or visual hallucinations (Mendez *et al.* 1990). The visual hallucinations commonly involve seeing small objects, insects or different colours, and often occur in the evening or at night when the light is dim. Auditory hallucinations may involve simple conversations or hearing voices or music.

Therefore, for the general population, psychotic features appear to be an integral part of DAD, particularly in advanced disease. For adults with ID and dementia, delusions and hallucinations are not often reported. Prasher (1997a) reviewed all reported cases of dementia in adults with DS up to that time. There were 86 cases in the final analysis. None of the individuals with dementia referred to the presence of any delusional phenomena, and only one individual referred to the possible presence of hallucinations. These findings suggest that psychotic phenomena of hallucinations and delusions are uncommon in adults with ID and dementia compared with the general population. This may be due to the fact that the underlying severity of ID does not allow the presentation of such symptoms. An alternative possibility is that such features may be present, but due to the underlying severity of ID they are not manifested. A third hypothesis is that such symptoms may be present and manifested, but are not detectable by clinicians. Further research in this area is required.

Treatment involves the use of antipsychotic medication and, where necessary, non-pharmacological interventions. The latter interventions may include improving sensory functions by using hearing aids and spectacles to prevent the misinterpretation of objects. Prominent features of hallucinations with a fluctuating mental state in a person with dementia may be indicative of Lewy body disease rather than DAD (Simard and Van Reekum 2001) (*see* Chapter 2).

Impairment in performance skills

Apraxia occurs when an individual has difficulty executing motor activities, even though they are able to move their arms and feet, and their understanding and sensory function (which may be other causes of inability to undertake activities) are unimpaired. It is a common symptom associated with DAD in the general population (Lorenzo-Otero 2001). Apraxia can present as difficulties with dressing, washing, feeding and mobility. The impairment in praxis skills increases as the course of the dementia progresses. Simple assessments can be undertaken as part of the initial clinical review. For example, if an individual is asked to wave goodbye, or shake hands, or put their hands above their head, failure to do so may indicate the presence of dyspraxia. More formal tests are available, in particular the Test of Praxis (Dalton *et al.* 1999), which was designed specifically to assess praxis skills in adults with ID. Dalton and his colleagues have demonstrated that in adults with DS and DAD, impairment in praxis follows the decline in cognitive skills (Dalton and Fedor 1998; Dalton *et al.* 1999).

Individuals may present with an inability to recognise familiar objects, such as a pen, a watch or a tie, in the presence of normal vision. In severe cases, examples of individuals who were unable to recognise family members or their own reflection have been reported.

Impairment of adaptive behaviour

With impairements in cognition and disturbance in emotion and behaviour, it is to be expected that DAD would also impact on adaptive behaviour (Zigman *et al.* 2002). A person with ID who develops dementia may only give rise to significant concern when there is a deterioration of their social and occupational skills, rather than when there is only intellectual impairment. Difficulties with dressing, bathing, feeding, helping with home-based activities or maintaining occupational activities can occur. Performance in these skills will have deteriorated from the person's previous level of functioning, and will deteriorate further as the process of DAD continues. The nature and severity of the impairment will vary with the individual, the degree of carer support and the environment, but generally the decline in adaptive behaviour is pervasive, and is present in a number of situations. Standardised rating scales are now available (*see* Chapter 5) for assessing the deterioration in adaptive behaviour.

A decline in adaptive behaviour in older adults with DS who develop dementia has been demonstrated by a number of cross-sectional longitudinal studies (for a review of studies, see Prasher 1998). Changes in adaptive behaviour have recently been demonstrated to be a screening measure for DAD in adults with DS (Prasher *et al.* 2004), and can also be used as an outcome measure in drug trials of anti-dementia therapy (Prasher *et al.* 2002b).

Mobility

Poor mobility in older adults with DAD can lead to an increase in falls and fractures, and an increased rate of admission to long-term facilities (Sattin 1992). Although the majority of falls do not lead to any serious injury or attendance at the Accident and Emergency department, approximately 5% of falls are associated with fractures. Bassiony *et al.* (2004) found that falls had occurred in 7.4% of patients in the general population with DAD during the last 2 weeks. Self-concern about mobility and increased anxiety about the possibility of falling and sustaining a fracture can lead to psychological problems such as loss of confidence, general anxiety and increased dependence on carers. Although mobility problems are usually associated with moderate and severe dementia, problems can still arise in the early stage of the disorder.

Adults with ID and DAD are particularly susceptible to falls. The greater the severity of cognitive problems, the greater is the risk of fractures and falls. For adults in the ID population the high risk of seizures associated with DAD, as well as impaired vision and frequent use of sedative medication, further increase the risk of falls and fractures (Day 1987). The commonest fractures associated with dementia are hip and wrist fractures, which can be up to 10 times more likely to occur in people with DAD compared with those without dementia.

The management of impaired mobility involves a detailed assessment of the risk of falls together with a detailed investigation of contributing factors. Means of preventing falls and preventing fractures should be explored, and a detailed physiotherapy assessment and occupational therapy assessment should be undertaken. Changes to the environment may be necessary along with increased physical support to enable the mobility to be more stable.

Eating problems and weight loss

Severe eating difficulties (including feeding, swallowing, positioning and behavioural difficulties) and marked weight loss have been reported to occur in adults in

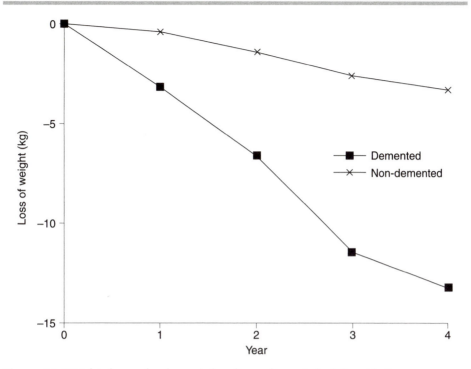

Figure 4.2 Weight change for demented and non-demented adults with Down syndrome. This figure is based on the original that appeared as figure 1, p. 3 in Prasher VP, Metseagharun T and Haque S (2004) Weight loss in adults with Down syndrome and with dementia in Alzheimer's disease. *Res Dev Disabil.* **25**: 1–7.

the general population with DAD (Wang *et al.* 2004) and in older adults with DS (Prasher *et al.* 2004) (*see* Figure 4.2). Associated with poor nutrition there may be secondary symptoms of general weakness, loss of muscle strength, mood changes, susceptibility to infection, episodes of aspirated pneumonia and an increased risk of death. Vitamin deficiency may further impact on cognitive function.

Dysphagia (swallowing difficulties due to oral and/or pharyngeal dysfunction) is common in DAD, particularly in the advanced stages of the dementia. This may be due to a combination of neurological, structural and psychological factors. Severe dysphagia will lead to malnutrition and marked weight loss, and can be a cause of considerable carer stress

Weight loss is particularly associated with end-stage DAD, although occasionally it may present before a diagnosis of DAD is made. Weight loss is a sign of malnutrition due to decreased calorie intake and difficulties in feeding oneself and/or swallowing food. Weight loss has been reported to predict mortality among adults in the general population with DAD (White *et al.* 1998). Weight loss in adults with DAD may be due to any of the following factors:

1 reduced food intake
2 increased body energy requirements
3 malabsorption of nutrients
4 changes in appetite
5 current medical disorders.

Little information is available about the management of weight loss and feeding problems in adults with ID who develop DAD. A detailed assessment of malnutrition and in particular the ability to swallow should be undertaken by a speech and language therapist with a view to improving calorie intake, maintaining weight and preventing aspiration pneumonia. Diet supplementation, help with feeding and carer advice and support can maintain good physical health. In end-stage dementia, tube feeding via a gastrostomy may be necessary, but as yet it has not been conclusively demonstrated that this has long-term significant benefits (Wang *et al.* 2004). Death due to aspiration pneumonia following repeated episodes of choking (due to the reduced level of consciousness, dysphagia and loss of gag reflux) is not uncommon (Kalia 2003).

Incontinence

Epidemiological studies would suggest a high prevalence of urinary and faecal incontinence in adults with dementia, both in the general population and in older adults with ID (Lai and Williams 1989; Evenhuis 1990; Schultz-Lampel 2003). Prevalence rates of up to 90% have been reported for adults with DAD. Regrettably, urinary and/or faecal incontinence is often given little attention as part of the clinical assessment and management (McCarthy and Mullan 1996). However, it can cause considerable psychological and social distress both to the affected person and to their carers. There may be an association with other urinary symptoms, such as frequency, urgency and nocturia.

There is limited information on the most appropriate management of incontinence in adults with ID who have dementia. A detailed history from carers, physical examination and necessary investigations should be part of the management plan, and a search for treatable causes of urinary tract symptoms should be undertaken. A urinary tract infection, faecal impaction, diabetes and side-effects of medication are common causes.

The management of urinary incontinence should involve specialist care (e.g. by a urinary incontinence nurse) and may include a number of behavioural techniques, medication (e.g. tricyclic antidepressants) or the use of appliances (e.g. incontinence pads or pants). General management measures with regard to fluid intake, bowel function and maintaining mobility can be beneficial. Regular toileting and a review of the use of laxatives should be undertaken. Secondary medical disorders associated with incontinence (e.g. urinary tract infections, perianal rash, pressure sores, emotional distress) should be treated. Incontinence can cause considerable stress to carers and can increase the risk of institutionalisation.

Seizures

Late-onset seizures are associated with DAD in the general population (Mendez *et al.* 1994; Hesdorffer *et al.* 1996) and are reported to occur in 15–25% of cases. Among the general population seizures are usually present in late-stage DAD, although they are more common in younger adults with DAD. Among the ID population, onset of seizures is also frequently reported to occur in adults with DS who develop DAD (Lai and Williams 1989; Evenhuis 1990). Lott and Lai (1982) reported generalised seizures in 9 of 15 DS patients with dementia. Wisniewski *et al.* (1985) found that 6 of 7 patients with DS and advanced dementia developed seizures. The prevalence of seizures can be up to 90% of DS adults with DAD, which is markedly higher than the prevalence for the general population.

Not infrequently seizures may be the first presenting feature to suggest an underlying dementing process. Generalised, partial and myoclonic seizures have been reported. An association between myoclonus and DAD in adults with DS has been reported (Blumbergs *et al.* 1981; Good and Howard 1982; Moller *et al.* 2001). However, further research is necessary to confirm the importance of this association. Seizures in elderly people with ID can be due to the initiation or cessation of psychotropic medication, and onset of seizures in adults with DS and DAD treated with anticholinesterase inhibitors has been reported (Prasher *et al.* 2002b).

Prasher and Corbett (1993) investigated life expectancy in adults with DS who developed late-onset seizures. The mean life expectancy of 9 individuals who developed seizures (out of 11 individuals with DAD) was 1.5 years. The authors concluded that late-onset seizures were a poor prognostic sign, indicating a probable life expectancy for most adults with DS who develop DAD of only 3 years after the first seizure.

The management of seizures in older adults with ID is not very different to that in younger adults. Treatable causes (e.g. subdural haematoma) should be investigated, and the type and severity of seizures should also be determined. Antiepileptic medication should be started at a low dosage and increased gradually. Carers will need to monitor closely both side-effects of medication and possible fractures associated with falls and post-ictal confusion. There is no clinical consensus as to which drugs should be used in individuals with an underlying dementing process, but the newer anticonvulsants may be more suitable.

Extrapyramidal features

Extrapyramidal features are common in adults with DAD in the general population (Mangone 2004). Virtually all prevalence-based studies of dementia in adults with DS have reported a high prevalence of extrapyramidal symptoms (see above). Vieregge *et al.* (1991) studied neurological signs in 54 demented and non-demented patients with DS, and found that of 14 patients who had dementia, five exhibited extrapyramidal signs, mainly of the rigid hyperkinetic spectrum.

There have been occasional case reports of parkinsonian disease in people with DS (Brandel *et al.* 1994). Bodhireddy *et al.* (1994) reported the case of a 40-year-old patient with DS and dementia and marked parkinsonian features. Whether these individuals have DAD which is associated with parkinsonian features, or Parkinson's disease, requires further investigation.

Sleep disturbance

An important feature of DAD is the disturbance of the sleep cycle. Sleep disturbance has been reported in up to 60% of adults in the general population, and is common in adults with ID who have DAD (Vitiello and Borson 2001; Bliwise 2004). There is a decrease in rapid eye movement (REM) sleep. Patients have difficulty in falling asleep, and can arise in the early hours believing that it is time to get up – to the point where they may get dressed and have breakfast or attempt to leave the home. Conversely, they may begin to sleep for long hours during the day. Sleep disturbance is associated with increased severity of DAD. Wandering at night may be associated with sleeplessness. In the general population, long-term evidence would suggest that up to 70% of individuals with dementia could have sleep problems (Cacabelos *et al.* 1996). Sleep disturbance may be directly associated with a disruption of the sleep cycle of a person with dementia, or it may be secondary to a psychiatric disorder (e.g. underlying depression). Disturbance of sleep, particularly when it disturbs the sleep of carers as well, is of considerable concern. The safety of the individual when they are unable to sleep and then begin to wander at night should be assessed.

Other associated features

Poor judgement and reduced insight are common findings in people with dementia. The person him- or herself may be unaware of the deterioration in intellectual and social functioning, or may appear vague and unresponsive during the interview. People with dementia may even participate in dangerous activities. Another common feature of DAD is wandering (Algase 1999), which involves aimless walking from one area to another, and can take place in the day or night. This may reflect the person's spatial disorientation.

Summary

Overall, the presentation of DAD in adults with ID is not too dissimilar to that seen in the general population. Due to the underlying cognitive impairment, some differences are seen, particularly in the presentation of early memory loss and perceptual change (e.g. delusions and hallucinations), but the insidious decline in cognitive functioning, loss of adaptive behaviour and development of associated physical features appear to occur in both populations. Any individual with ID who develops DAD will most probably present with some but not all of the features described above. The presenting psychopathology will be influenced by both genetic and environmental factors, the underlying cause of ID, age of onset, the severity of ID, and the carers' threshold for continuing to manage the patient. Certain symptoms may at certain times be of more concern. For example, in the early stages memory loss may be of most concern, but in the later stages immobility and faecal and urinary incontinence may cause the most distress. Further research is needed to establish the full picture of dementia in the different populations of adults with ID, further longitudinal studies are required to observe the natural progression and course of DAD, and further research is needed to determine the possible prodromal symptoms that may mark the onset of DAD.

Chapter 5

Assessment of dementia

Introduction

The clinical assessment and diagnosis of dementia in adults with intellectual disability (ID) have been the focus of considerable research over the last 30 years. However, the accurate diagnosis of dementia in Alzheimer's disease (DAD) in adults with ID, particularly in the early stages, remains difficult. It is still fraught with a high risk of inaccurate diagnosis or missed diagnosis. Inadequate assessments may fail to detect early memory and cognitive changes. Lack of understanding of the differential diagnosis for intellectual decline in older adults can lead to a premature and inaccurate diagnosis of DAD. There are several important reasons why an early diagnosis should be made (*see* Box 5.1).

Box 5.1 Importance of an early diagnosis of dementia

Reversible medical causes, such as depression and thyroid disease, can be identified and treated.

A correct diagnosis of DAD makes it possible to explain to carers and families what is happening.

It enables the affected person and their carers to plan future care.

Psychiatric treatment can be initiated, which may include psychological therapy and anti-dementia medication.

Carer support/education can be provided.

The dementia assessment

The cornerstone of the assessment is a detailed clinical appraisal with supporting evidence from neuropsychological and medical investigations. A detailed comprehensive assessment for DAD is time-consuming, particularly in older adults with ID. Because of its complexity this assessment should be conducted by a specialist, not by the general practitioner or by professionals who lack the appropriate training. The majority of the initial assessment process should be undertaken in the individual's own home. This ensures that the patient is relaxed, their environment can be assessed, and a number of carers can be interviewed. Memory clinics are now available for the general population, and are being established in the field of ID. These clinics are an alternative venue for the initial assessments, and have the advantage of allowing neuropsychological and medical investigations to take place on the same visit.

Whenever possible the comprehensive assessment of a person with ID for dementia should be undertaken by the multi-disciplinary team (MDT). This would include a psychiatrist specialising in ID, a clinical psychologist, a community nurse and a social worker as the core team. The involvement of other individuals, such as the general practitioner, occupational therapist, physiotherapist, pharmacist and district nurse, should be considered in order to provide support and information with regard to specific clinical needs. It is not possible for all professionals to be present at an initial joint assessment. Practically it may be necessary for a series of separate consultations to take place, with a subsequent review of all information at an MDT meeting.

After all of the individual professional assessments have been undertaken, the MDT will find that patients usually fall into one of the following six groups:

1 well – with no evidence of intellectual decline
2 well – but showing age-associated functional decline (normal ageing)
3 showing intellectual decline due to a physical disorder (e.g. thyroid dysfunction, sensory loss)
4 showing intellectual decline due to a psychiatric disorder (e.g. depression)
5 showing degenerative dementia (e.g. Alzheimer's disease)
6 miscellaneous group (delirium, drug toxicity).

The assessment process for diagnosing dementia is complex (*see* Figure 5.1). The first aim of the assessment process is always to determine where there has been intellectual decline (and decline in adaptive behaviour). This can be complicated in the case of adults with ID living in care establishments where different staff may be looking after a given person. Caregivers may not detect intellectual

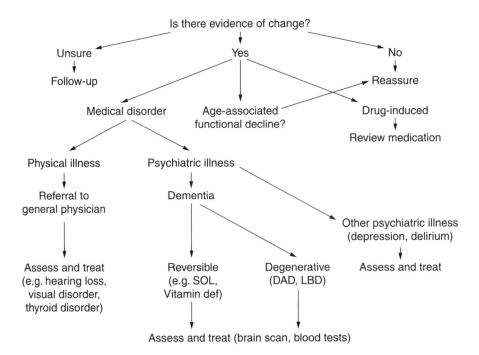

Figure 5.1 Assessment process in diagnosing dementia.

decline over time, or if they do, they may assume that it is part of the underlying ID or due to ageing *per se*. Furthermore, carers may often not have the necessary knowledge of the different physical and psychiatric illnesses and how they present. For example, the misplacing of items may be attributed to the person with ID 'just being difficult'. Therefore, for a significant group of individuals, repeat assessments over time will be the only reliable way in which clinicians will become aware of presenting psychopathology that is suggestive of an underlying dementing process.

Once a change in intellectual and/or adaptive behaviour has been established, the next step is to determine whether the change is due to age-associated functional decline (normal ageing) or to an underlying physical or psychiatric illness. As mentioned earlier, it may be difficult to establish whether psychological change has occurred, and follow-up over time (with formal assessments) may be the only way to detect absolute change.

If the change in intellectual functioning is thought to be greater than that which would be expected as part of normal ageing, and a diagnosis of a possible medical disorder has been made, then it is important to determine the underlying cause, in particular identifying treatable causes. The exclusion of physical disorders as a cause of intellectual impairment/decline in adaptive behaviour is usually possible by means of a routine physical examination and standard investigatory tests. These tests would include the following:

1 blood tests to exclude a whole range of biochemical and haematological disorders (especially thyroid dysfunction)
2 hearing and vision assessments to rule out significant hearing loss or visual impairment
3 electroencephalography or a brain scan (CT or MRI) to exclude a space-occupying lesion.

The exclusion of a psychiatric disorder (e.g. depression) requires a specialist neuropsychiatric assessment. Depression can mimic dementia and does commonly occur alongside the latter. If there are concerns that a depressive illness may be present, a trial course of antidepressant therapy and appropriate follow-up over time may be an appropriate initial form of treatment. Delirium is usually of rapid onset with a fluctuating course, usually worse at night, with an impaired conscious level. There may be marked mood swings, restlessness and agitation, with prominent visual illusions, hallucinations and paranoid ideas. If delirium is suspected, further investigations including electroencephalography and a review of medication should be undertaken.

Dementia assessment process

If a dementia assessment is to be successful, rapport needs to be established with both the patient and the informants. A non-threatening, friendly interview technique needs to be used. Once rapport has been established and the relevant background information has been obtained from carers, a semi-structured interview should be conducted with the patient. It is important to assess the individual's underlying severity of ID, as this will determine their level of ability with regard to understanding and answering questions. Figure 5.2 shows the usual steps of a dementia work-up.

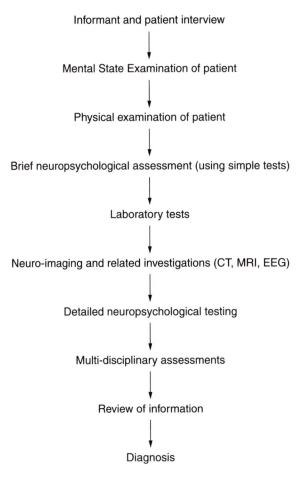

Figure 5.2 Dementia work-up (some aspects of the process may be omitted).

Psychiatric interview

It is imperative that a psychiatric interview is undertaken in a trusting and confiding environment in which accurate and relevant information about the patient's current problems can be elicited. Furthermore, an assessment of aetiological factors, examination of the patient's mental state, assessment of the impact on the patient and carers, and of the reliability of carer informants, and determination of a diagnostic formulation are all important aspects of the interview. A systematic assessment should be undertaken that covers several areas, many of which may appear to be irrelevant, but all of which provide valuable information for making an accurate diagnosis of DAD and subsequently determining the most appropriate treatment plan.

Presenting problem

The majority of older adults with ID, because of the underlying severity of ID, are unable to provide detailed information about decline in memory or language, or

Table 5.1 Important areas to ask about when interviewing informants

Area	Specific problem
General features	Time of onset of problems, duration, initial symptoms, general course. Impact on carers and other members of household
Cognitive symptoms	Memory, speech and language, visuo-spatial and perceptual changes
Neuropsychiatric symptoms	Personality change, behavioural change, loss of volition, mood changes, psychotic phenomena, eating habits, sleep pattern changes, sexual behavioural problems, aggression, wandering, lability of mood
Activities of daily living	Dressing, washing, feeding, day care activities, domestic activities
Physical symptoms	Onset of seizures, incontinence, weight loss, stiffness

about failure to participate in social activities as well as previously. It is important that an informant is available to give detailed information, particularly with regard to sensitive issues, and to provide information about the impact of the dementia. Ideally the informant should be someone who has known the individual for a long time and has been involved in caring for him or her over the last few years. If this is not the case, it is good practice for a family member to be present together with the present carer.

A standard medical interview will determine when the symptoms started, in which order, and how they have progressed during the course of the dementing process. Important factors that either alleviate or worsen the dementia should be determined. Specific areas that need to be assessed during the informant's interview are listed in Table 5.1.

Family history

Although this is uncommon, it is important to assess for a possible family history of dementia, including the age of onset, cause of death and type of dementia. This may prove difficult in the case of older adults with ID who are being cared for in residential facilities, but where possible family information should be obtained. Information about other hereditary disorders that may impact on health (e.g. a family history of diabetes or strokes) should be elicited.

Medical history

Any history of seizures, head injuries, strokes or any recent illness that has affected consciousness should be elicited. A past history of heart disease, thyroid disease or vitamin deficiency should be noted.

Psychiatric history

One of the commonest differential diagnoses of dementia in an elderly person with or without ID is depression. Is there a history of recurrent depressive episodes? Commonly associated symptoms of depression which should be assessed are concerned with change in affect (low mood, tiredness, apathy), biological features of depression (sleep deterioration, loss of appetite, loss of weight, early-morning wakening) and a recent history of behavioural problems. Paranoid ideas and hallucinations may sometimes be present. (For further information about depressive symptomatology, *see* Chapter 4.)

Medication

All medication (prescribed or otherwise) should be reviewed as a cause of intellectual decline or as a cause that could impair intellectual functioning further. Medication that is no longer taken but was prescribed previously should also be considered, as many of the drugs that are used in the ID population can have chronic effects many years after they have been stopped.

Social circumstances

Where the person is living is an important factor. Are they living alone, with their own family, or in an institution? The type of information that is obtained will be influenced by the person's place of residence. For example, a disturbed sleep pattern may have a greater impact in the family home, whereas paranoia may lead to episodes of aggression when there are many other people in close proximity. Evidence for a decline in several settings is important. Do particular symptoms cause particular concern in different settings?

General review

A general review of physical and psychiatric health is important to exclude other causes of decline and to help to determine the actual cause. Is there a history of recent hospital admissions? Is there evidence of a mental illness (e.g. schizophrenia)? Has there been a recent bereavement? Does the intellectual impairment fluctuate?

Physical symptoms

A history of associated physical features of dementia, such as incontinence, impaired mobility, weight loss and seizures, should be taken. The chronological order is important and will help to determine the type and severity of the dementia.

Mental State Examination

The Mental State Examination is an appraisal of the mental health of the patient by direct and indirect assessments. It begins the moment the patient walks into the room and finishes when they leave. The different components of a standard Mental State Examination are listed in Box 5.2.

Box 5.2 Different domains of the Mental State Examination

Appearance. Dress, posture, self-hygiene, mobility, behaviour, psychomotor activity (agitated, slow movements).

Mood. Depressed, anxious, irritable, angry, frightened, labile, apathetic.

Communication. Quality, quantity and rate of speech, aphasia, response to questions.

Perceptions. Hallucinations – usually auditory 'voices', but can be visual, olfactory or tactile. Delusions – may be persecutory, grandiose, jealous, etc.

Thought process (determined by underlying level of ID). Coherent, answers questions appropriately, delusional, has suicidal thoughts or thoughts about harming others.

Insight (self-awareness of illness). Lack of awareness of one's own illness.

Personality change. Aggressive, irritable, paranoid, apathetic, mood changes, passive.

Rituals. Repeated action such as checking or cleaning.

Cognition. Orientation, registration, memory, recall, language.

The Mental State Examination is ongoing while information is being obtained from informants and while other assessments are being conducted (e.g. physical examination). The examination can support the information given during the interview and can help to focus the questions that are directed to carers. For example, if the patient looks unhappy and is tearful, a greater emphasis would be given to questions related to depression when questioning the informant.

Some aspects of the Mental State Examination do require patient cooperation, particularly when eliciting delusions and hallucinations. Caution is needed if cooperation is poor or not forthcoming. The aim of the cognition assessment is to determine the evidence for cognitive impairment. A number of neuropsychological tests are available to formalise this process (see section on neuropsychological tests).

Physical examination

A general physical examination should be performed. Particular attention should be given to the assessment of hearing and vision. For example, the development of cataracts may have led to loss of skills. The presence of heart disease and/or hypertension may suggest vascular dementia. Extrapyramidal symptoms (e.g. a pill-rolling tremor, or rigidity) may suggest Lewy body dementia. Weight loss should be monitored.

Laboratory tests

Routine laboratory tests and neuroimaging investigations can detect underlying causes of dementia and can also exclude causes of intellectual decline, enabling a more reliable diagnosis of DAD to be made. Chapter 6 reviews the different investigations used to diagnose DAD.

Neuropsychological tests

Historically, psychological testing has played a major part in the diagnosis of dementia. As there are no normative total population standards for many neuropsychological tests, either for the general population or in particular for the ID population, abnormal performance has often been determined by comparison with a 'normal' control group matched for age, sex, educational level, ID and other factors. A score falling in the lowest fifth percentile of an individual's 'normal' control group has often been designated as 'abnormal'. Progressive worsening of the psychopathology of the dementia can be established by comparison with previous performance on neuropsychological testing.

Different neuropsychological tests of cognitive ability have been used to investigate intellectual decline in the ID population. These include intelligence tests (Nakamura 1961; Hewitt et al. 1985; Fenner et al. 1987), delayed match-to-sample tests of short-term memory (Dalton and Crapper-McLachlan 1984; Dalton and Wisniewski 1990), visual memory tests (Dalton and McMurray 1995), the tabletop spatial location test (a test of the location of familiar objects in space) and the dyspraxia test (Dalton 1996). Researchers have consistently demonstrated that older adults with DS perform less well than younger subjects in many areas of cognitive functioning (Owens et al. 1971; Dalton et al. 1974; Thase et al. 1984). The authors have therefore argued that such tests may be able to detect cognitive deterioration as part of a dementing process. Haxby (1989), using a battery of neuropsychological tests administered to 10 adults with DS over the age of 35 years and 19 younger adults with DS, found that the DS adults with dementia had global neuropsychological deficits as indicated by significant differences on all functions tested. These included orientation, registration, attention, calculation and recall. The one exception was some simple language functions. In contrast, elderly adults without dementia had a selective pattern of neuropsychological reduction relative to young adults. Ability to retain new long-term memories and visuo-spatial construction were consistently diminished, whereas immediate memory span and language were not affected.

Neuropsychological testing has an important role to play in the detection of DAD in older adults with ID (Silverman et al. 2004). Cognitive deficits are undoubtedly present in a person with ID who develops dementia. To date, different tests have been employed, often on small samples, with preselected subjects who complete the tests, often involving cross-sectional studies with non-ID subjects as controls, non-validated criteria for dementia and no screening for underlying causes of test failure. Few population-based studies have been undertaken to investigate the applicability of neuropsychological testing to individuals with ID with a wide age range, a wide range of intellectual levels and coexisting medical disorders. Neuropsychological testing aids the clinical dementia work-up by formally documenting the level of cognitive skills, reliably monitoring change over time, providing outcome measures for pharmacological treatment and determining the degree of capacity. Detailed administration of a test battery can be time-consuming (e.g. it may take up to 2–3 hours) and tiring for the examiner, patient and carer. Appropriate training in the administration and interpretation of scores is important. The possibility of misdiagnosis or inappropriate diagnosis of dementia is a cause for concern.

The implementation of existing tests that are used in the non-ID population (e.g. the Mini Mental State Examination) is inappropriate for people with severe and profound ID due to the 'floor effect'. Simple questions such as 'Do you know what day it is?' or 'Do you know how old you are?' are often answered incorrectly by adults with ID even when they are 'well'.

Furthermore, many tests usually require the patient to have good communication and language skills, reasonable dexterity in performing actions, and good vision and hearing for comprehending instructions, and it is assumed that there will be no disturbed behaviour and a reasonable amount of cooperation. The patient's level of intellectual functioning before the onset of dementia may not be known. Poor performance on any test items may therefore be due to the underlying ID, secondary to associated phenotypic behaviours and/or associated health morbidity, rather than due to the onset of DAD.

Neuropsychological tests for dementia in the general population

Numerous assessment scales are available for use in the elderly general population to aid the psychiatric assessment of dementia (*see* Table 5.2).

The most commonly used assessment instrument in the general population is the Mini Mental State Examination (MMSE) (Folstein *et al.* 1975), which has been widely used over the last 30 years. The MMSE is a 30-point scale that assesses areas such as orientation, memory, registration, attention, calculation, language and constructional ability. It is relatively simple and quick to administer (5 to 10 minutes), and provides a high degree of sensitivity and specificity for dementia. The maximum possible score is 30 points, but if there is severe visual impairment, areas that require good vision can be skipped and a total of 27 points can be used. However, if severe hearing loss is present, the MMSE cannot be used. The test does depend on the patient's ability to comprehend and respond to verbal instructions. It is generally accepted that a score of less than 24 strongly suggests dementia. However, as with many other screening instruments, other conditions (e.g. depression, intellectual disability, stroke) can lead to a low score suggestive of dementia.

Other popular tests that are widely used in the general population are the Abbreviated Mental Test Score (AMTS) (Qureshi and Hodkinson 1974) and the Clock Drawing Test (Brodaty and Moore 1997). The AMTS is derived from the Mental Test Score, which was in turn derived from the Blessed Dementia Scale. The ATMS is a 10-item scale that is used to screen for cognitive impairment. A score of 7 or lower suggests a degree of dementia. Like the MMSE, it requires the patient to have good communication and language skills, and test failure can be due to other psychiatric disorders. The Clock Drawing Test tests the patient's ability to draw a clock face with the hours numbered and the hands indicating a particular time. A score is given depending on the accuracy of the clock face, the order of the numbers and the position of the hands. Usually a misshapen clock will give a general idea that there is something wrong. The Clock Drawing Test assesses a number of domains, including memory, language, comprehension, visuo-spatial skills, visual motor skills, fine motor skills and visual fields.

Table 5.2 Psychiatric measures used to detect DAD in the general population

Assessment scale	Main indication
Global assessment	
CDR (Clinical Dementia Rating)	Global measure of dementia
BPRS (Brief Psychiatric Rating Scale)	Global psychiatric symptoms
CAMDEX (Cambridge Mental Disorders of the Elderly Examination)	Diagnosis of dementia
Neuropsychological assessment	
MMSE (Mini Mental State Examination)	Screening for dementia
AMTS (Abbreviated Mental Test Score)	Screening for dementia
ADAS (Alzheimer's Disease Assessment Scale)	Assessment of cognition
Clock-Drawing Test	Screening for dementia
Neuropsychiatric assessment	
BEHAVE-AD (Behavioural Symptoms in Alzheimer's Disease)	Behavioural symptoms
NPI (Neuropsychiatric Inventory)	Psychopathology
MOUSEPAD (Manchester and Oxford Universities Scale for the Psychopathological Assessment of Dementia)	Psychiatric change
RAGE (Rating Scale for Aggressive Behaviour in the Elderly)	Aggressive behaviour
Activities of daily living	
ADL (Activities of Daily Living Index)	Daily living function
FAQ (Functional Activities Questionnaire)	Functional capacity
Caregiver assessments	
Burden Interview	Feelings of burden
Marital Intimacy Scale	Assessment of relationship with partner
Cornel Scale for Depression in Dementia	Diagnosis of depression in dementia

A more detailed neuropsychological assessment may be required after the initial clinical assessment and the use of screening tools. Neuropsychologists can provide a detailed assessment of the different intellectual domains, and can sometimes diagnose the onset of DAD before a clinician. Psychometric testing is particularly important in the early stages of DAD, but can also be used to monitor the progression of the disease or to measure the response to treatment. Furthermore, neuropsychologists can have an important role to play in the ongoing management of dementia, particularly in people with ID.

Neuropsychological tests for dementia in the ID population

For the ID population, there are a number of instruments available to aid the clinical assessment of dementia. These are listed in Table 5.3.

The principal screening instruments that have been used in the ID population are the Dementia Questionnaire for Mentally Retarded Persons (DMR) (Evenhuis *et al.* 1990, Evenhuis 1992), the Test for Severe Impairment (TSI) (Albert and Cohen 1992) and the Dementia Scale for Down Syndrome (DSDS) (Gedye 1995).

The DMR (Evenhuis *et al.* 1990) is a quick informant-based questionnaire designed to be completed by caregivers. This instrument has 8 subscales (short-term memory, long-term memory, spatial and temporal orientation, speech, practical skills, mood, activity and interests, and behavioural disturbance). The different items can be summed to give the Sum of Cognitive Scores (SCS) (short-term memory, long-term memory, and spatial and temporal orientation) and the Sum of Social Scores (SOS) (speech, practical skills, mood, activity and interests, and behavioural disturbance). Cut-off scores that are determined by the severity of ID are used to detect the presence of dementia. Although the author reported results for single cross-sectional scores, Evenhuis (1996) recommended that score changes over time would be the most valid criterion, as single-assessment cut-off scores could be inaccurate (Prasher 1997b; Strydom and Hassiotis 2003). Prasher (1997b) found that with modification of the cut-off scores and the criteria used, the DMR questionnaire did have good diagnostic validity for dementia.

The TSI (Albert and Cohen 1992) is a brief neuropsychological test that takes approximately 10 minutes to administer. It minimises the use of language, and can be used across a wide spectrum of people with ID. It has six subsections, namely motor function, language, comprehension, delayed memory, general knowledge and conceptualisation. Cosgrave *et al.* (1998) investigated the use of the TSI to assess dementia in 60 adults with DS, and found that this instrument was a useful performance-based measure for assessing cognitive decline in older adults with DS.

The DSDS (Gedye 1995) assesses cognitive deterioration, principally in people with moderate to profound ID. It is an informant-based test, and requires a psychologist to interview two informants. There are 60 questions, which divide the dementia into early, middle and late stages. A number of researchers have assessed the DSDS (Deb and Braganza 1999; Huxley *et al.* 2000; Temple *et al.* 2001; Strydom and Hassiotos 2003). Conflicting results have been published with regard to the sensitivity and specificity of the DSDS in screening for dementia in people with ID.

Das *et al.* (1995) investigated the use of the Dementia Rating Scale (DRS) to detect DAD in adults with DS. A total of 46 subjects with DS were studied together

Table 5.3 Instruments for assessing dementia in the ID population

Assessment scale	Main indication
Global assessment	
DMR (Dementia Questionnaire for Mentally Retarded Persons)	Screening for dementia
CAMDEX-Ds	Diagnosis of dementia
Neuropsychological assessment	
DSDS (Dementia Scale for Down Syndrome)	Screening for dementia
TSI (Test for Severe Impairment)	Screening for dementia
Early Signs of Dementia Checklist	Screening for dementia
Prudhoe Cognitive Functioning Test	Screening for dementia
BPT (Brief Praxis Test)	Praxia
Neuropsychiatric assessment	
DSMSE (Down Syndrome Mental State Examination)	Dementia symptoms
PRIMA (Psychopathology Instrument for Mentally Retarded Adults)	Psychiatric problems
Activities of daily living	
Vineland Adaptive Behaviour Scales	Adaptive behaviour
AAMD-ABS Part I and II (AAMD-Adaptive Behaviour Scale I and II)	Adaptive behaviour
ABC (Aberrant Behaviour Checklist)	Behaviour disturbance
ABDQ (Adaptive Behaviour Dementia Questionnaire)	Screening for DAD

with 54 non-DS subjects with ID. Only five individuals with DS were aged 50 years or over. The DRS measured five specific cognitive abilities, namely attention, initiation/preservation, construction, conceptualisation and memory. Significantly lower scores were detected by the scale for all five cognitive abilities in individuals with DS aged 50 years or over. The authors argued that the DRS was therefore a valid test for dementia in the DS population.

Prasher *et al.* (2004) recently published an analysis of 5-year consecutive adaptive behaviour data. Using these data the authors developed a research-based clinical screening tool for dementia in Alzheimer's disease (DAD) in adults with DS (ABDQ). This is a 15-item questionnaire, completed by carers, which is used to detect changes in adaptive behaviour. The scale has good reliability and validity, with an overall accuracy of 92%. Unlike other instruments designed to screen for dementia, the ABDQ was designed specifically to screen for DAD.

Diagnostic criteria for dementia in Alzheimer's disease (DAD)

Historically, DAD was diagnosed by clinicians and researchers on the basis of the presence of a number of ill-defined symptoms and signs without reference to a given standard. In the 1960s the Mental Health Programme of the World Health Organization began to develop a diagnostic and classification system for all mental disorders, including dementia. By the late 1970s there was growing international interest in the accurate diagnosis of DAD and in the need to differentiate between DAD and other forms of dementia. In 1992 the tenth revision of the *International Classification of Diseases (ICD-10)* was published (World Health Organization 1992).

Dementia in Alzheimer's disease is not a well-defined single disease entity, but is made up of a variety of aetiological, pathological and clinical processes. It is even more complex in adults with ID due to the underlying severity of intellectual impairment, comorbid health disorders and lack of reliable background information. Sometimes, although an accurate diagnosis of DAD is difficult, such a diagnosis is important because it allows the most appropriate treatment plan to be implemented, treatable causes to be identified, preventive measures to be put in place, and international research to be standardised. Alzheimer's disease is principally a neuropathological diagnosis characterised by a high prevalence of senile plaques and neurofibrillary tangles. However, a diagnostic brain biopsy is not ethically acceptable when a person is alive, and therefore a clinical diagnosis of DAD must be made. As there is no highly sensitive and specific biological marker for the disease, a cluster of clinical symptoms and signs is used to make a clinical diagnosis. This cluster of clinical features must be characteristic of DAD in order to distinguish it from other forms of dementia. For the general population there are four widely used systems of diagnostic criteria for diagnosing DAD (*see* Box 5.3).

Box 5.3 Systems of diagnostic criteria for DAD

Tenth revision of the *International Classification of Diseases (ICD-10)* (World Health Organization 1992)

Fourth edition of the *Diagnostic and Statistical Manual of Mental Disorders (DSM-IV)* (American Psychiatric Association 1994)

National Institute of Neurological and Communicative Disorders and Stroke/Alzheimer's Disease and Related Disorders Association (NINCDS-ADRDA) Work Group Criteria (McKann *et al.* 1984)

The Consortium to Establish a Registry for Alzheimer's Disease Criteria (Morris *et al.* 1989)

These systems do show similarities, but there are also important differences (*see* Table 5.4). Furthermore, it must be borne in mind that the accuracy of these

Table 5.4 Features of *ICD-10* and *DSM-IV* criteria

	ICD-10 criteria	*DSM-IV criteria*
Memory decline	+	+
Cognitive impairment	+	−
Aphasia	−	+
Apraxia	−	+
Agnosia	−	+
Impairment in daily activities	+	−
Social or occupational impairment	−	+
Decline from a previous level of functioning	+	+
Insidious onset	+	+
Slow deterioration	+	−
Ongoing progressive deterioration	−	+
Absence of systemic disorder	+	+
Absence of sudden onset	+	−
Absence of focal neurological signs	+	−

criteria for diagnosing clinical DAD is of the order of 80% (Tierney *et al.* 1988; Galasko *et al.* 1994). Therefore their accuracy for detecting DAD in adults with ID will presumably be much lower.

The *ICD-10* criteria (World Health Organization 1992) define DAD principally as a decline in memory and thinking which has a significant impact on personal activities of daily living. There is an insidious onset with slow deterioration, and there is an absence of other systemic or brain disease that can induce dementia and an absence of focal neurological signs. The duration of the above symptoms must be at least 6 months. The *DSM-IV* criteria (American Psychiatric Association 1994) define dementia of the Alzheimer's type as a disorder of multiple cognitive deficits manifested by both memory impairment and disturbances in at least one of the following areas: aphasia, apraxia, agnosia or executive functioning. As with the *ICD-10* criteria (World Health Organization 1992), such cognitive impairment should be severe enough to affect social and occupational functioning, with a significant decline from a previous level of functioning. There is a gradual onset with continuing decline. Other central nervous system conditions, systemic conditions and substance-induced conditions are excluded. The deficits are not due to delirium or any other major mental illness. According to *ICD-10* (World Health Organization 1992) and *DSM-IV* (American Psychiatric Association 1994) criteria, dementia due to Alzheimer's disease can be subdivided by the age of 65 years into 'early onset' or 'late onset'.

There are several problems with regard to the use of the above diagnostic systems. For example, they do not state how one detects or determines specific symptoms and signs (e.g. dysphasia or agnosia). Neurological symptoms such as incontinence, gait disturbance and seizures are not mentioned. Furthermore, the degree of memory loss and the degree of deterioration is often not stated. Overall, however, given the limitations of all the diagnostic criteria, they have improved the accuracy of a clinical diagnosis of DAD.

Although over the last 30 years diagnostic criteria have been developed for the general population in order to improve the accuracy of the clinical diagnosis of DAD, no such criteria have been developed specifically for the ID population. Clinicians have either used the same criteria as those employed for the general population, or modified these criteria and then applied them to adults with ID, or developed their own idiosyncratic diagnostic criteria. There are advantages and drawbacks for each method, but generally none of them have a sound research basis.

Summary

The assessment and diagnosis of dementia in people with ID continue to be the focus of international interest (Janicki *et al.* 1996). The assessment process is the same as that for the general population, although its implementation and the interpretation of findings are different. However, if the format of the process is followed, it is highly likely that as far as is possible an accurate clinical diagnosis of dementia and the underlying type of dementia will be made.

Aylward *et al.* (1997) published international guidelines on the diagnostic criteria for a diagnosis of dementia in the ID population, in an attempt to overcome the lack of available standardised assessments. These guidelines have yet to be fully implemented in clinical practice. Several screening tests for dementia and for DAD in adults with ID are available, but they are not diagnostic for DAD. There is still concern about the reliability and validity of these tests in detecting cognitive decline (e.g. of memory, orientation, attention span) and impairment of other intellectual functions (e.g. speech, comprehension, aphasia, apraxia), and in demonstrating accurately a decline in intellectual functioning (a prerequisite for dementia) in older people with a wide spectrum of underlying severity of ID.

It is probable that in contrast to the general population, which is more homologous, because of the greater variability in adults with ID no one neuropsychological test will be suitable for detecting DAD in all adults with ID. However, ongoing research is investigating the possibility of a biological marker being identified and used as a diagnostic measure for DAD. Until such a test becomes available, a detailed and conscientious clinical assessment remains the core process in the diagnosis of DAD in adults with ID.

Chapter 6

Investigations for dementia

Introduction

It remains a failing of professionals working in the field of intellectual disability (ID) that far too often a diagnosis of dementia, and particularly a diagnosis of dementia in Alzheimer's disease (DAD), is made without the appropriate investigations being undertaken. This is of particular concern because the features that are an essential part of a definite diagnosis according to *ICD-10* (World Health Organization 1992) or *DSM-IV* (American Psychiatric Association 1994) criteria for DAD require investigations to be undertaken and treatable causes of dementia excluded. A number of laboratory investigations are mandatory in the diagnosis of DAD, including haematological, biochemical and endocrinological assessments.

Electroencephalography remains the most widely available non-invasive test, but has in the last two decades been superseded by more sophisticated investigations. Computed tomography (CT) and nuclear magnetic resonance imaging (MRI) have resulted in a number of new developments that enable the structure of the brain to be investigated in detail. Single photon emission computed tomography (SPECT) and positron emission tomography (PET) have developed into tests that involve the application of quantitative tracer methodology to investigate cerebral function.

Brain imaging studies are usually less readily accessible by the ID population than by the general population. Whether such tests are undertaken depends upon the specific dementia profile. Evidence of a space-occupying lesion, or a recent history of head trauma, should lead to a brain imaging assessment. Brain scans assess brain structure and/or function for diagnostic patterns of abnormalities that correlate with clinical dementia.

The need for further investigations will need to be reviewed on a regular basis. For example, if brain scanning is not undertaken initially it may be required at a later date if deterioration is more rapid than expected, or if unexpected symptoms (e.g. hemiparesis) are manifested.

The possible causes of dementia were discussed in Chapter 2. In this chapter the investigations necessary to determine the type and cause of the dementia will be considered.

Laboratory tests

Laboratory tests are an essential part of the assessment of dementia, but sadly are often not undertaken. Standard tests that should be undertaken are listed in Table 6.1. These tests are particularly important during the initial assessment, although

Table 6.1 Essential laboratory tests in the assessment of dementia

Test	Conditions screened for by test
Haematological – full blood count (FBC)	Anaemia, macrocytosis, platelet disorder infections
Vitamin B_{12}, folate	Vitamin B_{12} or folate deficiency
Clinical chemistry (profile)	Electrolyte deficiency (e.g. hyponatraemia, hypocalcaemia)
Renal function (blood urea nitrogen (BUN), creatinine, urea)	Renal impairment
Liver function (albumin, alkaline phosphatase, aspartate transaminase, bilirubin)	Liver impairment
Glucose	Diabetes mellitus
Thyroid function (thyroxine, thyroid-stimulating hormone)	Hypothyroidism
Urate	Gout
Erythrocyte sedimentation rate (ESR)	Inflammatory disorders
Urinalysis	Urinary tract infection

they should be repeated on a regular basis even after the diagnosis of dementia has been confirmed. They exclude other causes of cognitive impairment (e.g. delirium), systemic endocrine disorders (e.g. thyroid disease, diabetes), and organ impairment and disease (e.g. of kidneys or liver), and can detect uncommon causes of dementia (e.g. vitamin B_{12} or folate deficiency).

Neurophysiological tests

Electrophysiological methods

Electroencephalography (EEG) recordings of patients with DAD in the general population can show increased slow-wave activity (an increase in theta- and delta-wave activity) (Saletu 1991; Knott *et al.* 2000; Jeong 2004). Therefore EEG recordings have been proposed as a potential tool to aid the clinical diagnosis of DAD. Furthermore, an EEG can help to distinguish between dementia and delirium, detect an associated seizure disorder and confirm organic brain pathology.

A number of studies have investigated an association between EEG abnormalities and DAD in adults with DS. Devinsky *et al.* (1990) studied 19 young adults (aged 19–37 years) and 9 older patients (aged 42–66 years) with DS, together with healthy controls from the general population. All patients with DS had trisomy 21 and were recruited from the community. Four of the older patients with DS had a clinical diagnosis of dementia. The EEG alpha background activity was normal in 13 (68%) and abnormal in 6 (32%) of the young adults with DS. The activity was normal in 5 (56%) and abnormal in 4 (44%) of the older patients with DS. All of the controls had normal background activity. All four individuals with both DS and dementia showed loss of alpha background activity and increased slow-wave activity. The authors concluded that these findings may be associated with dementia, but are probably a non-specific change associated with ageing.

Using a larger sample, Soininen *et al.* (1993) investigated EEG changes in 31 patients with DS compared with adults with DAD from the general population and age-matched non-demented controls from the general population. The mean age of the DS group was 35 years (range 21–60 years). All three groups were assessed by means of the Mini Mental State Examination (Folstein *et al.* 1975), together with a combination of neuropsychological tests of speech functioning, praxic functioning, visual functioning and recall. The researchers found an age-related decline in cortical functions and increased slowing of EEG activity in the DS group. This supported the view that an increase in EEG slow-wave activity was due to normal ageing rather than to a dementing disease process.

In contrast, however, Visser *et al.* (1996) investigated the use of EEG recordings to detect dementia in 197 adults with DS who were monitored for 5–8 years. Cognitive functioning was assessed twice per year using a Dutch version of the Cain–Levine Social Competence Rating Scale (Cain *et al.* 1963). A significant decline in cognitive function was seen in 29 subjects over the study period. In these subjects the dominant occipital rhythm became slower at the onset of the cognitive deterioration, and eventually disappeared with progression of the deterioration. The authors were more optimistic than previous researchers about the role of EEG measurements as a means of detecting DAD changes in adults with DS.

On balance, there does appear to be an increase in abnormalities in EEG recordings of brain function for people with DS as they age, and this seems to be even more marked in individuals with clinical dementia. Loss of alpha rhythm with an increase in theta rhythm and/or delta activity, similar to DAD in the general population, may be seen. However, the sensitivity and specificity for DAD in people with DS are likely to be low, and therefore although EEG recordings are an important part of the assessment of a person presenting with intellectual decline, they appear to have a limited role as a test for diagnosing DAD.

Evoked potentials

Because of the limited role of the standard EEG as a tool to aid the clinical diagnosis of DAD, researchers have subsequently modified the EEG assessment by using evoked potentials. These are a form of EEG that records brain-wave activity associated with sensory stimulation or other stimulatory events (auditory, somatosensory or visual). Auditory and visual evoked potentials have been most widely investigated.

Auditory evoked potentials

Several studies have been published that have reported a delay in latency and other abnormalities of the principal auditory evoked potential (P300) in adults from the general population with DAD (Williams *et al.* 1991; Olichney and Hillert 2004). Few studies to date have commented on the use of auditory evoked potentials to detect DAD in the DS population (Blackwood *et al.* 1988; Muir *et al.* 1988).

Blackwood *et al.* (1988) conducted a study designed to assess the role of the auditory P300 response as a measure of the onset of dementia in adults with DS.

Auditory evoked potentials were recorded from 89 individuals with DS aged 16–66 years. A control group consisting of 29 age-matched individuals with ID and fragile X syndrome and 89 age-matched controls from the general population controls was also tested. Clinical psychological testing found evidence of dementia in 16 individuals with DS and in none of the individuals with fragile X syndrome. There was a marked increase in P300 latency starting at around 37 years of age in the DS population, but not in the other two groups. In controls the effect of age on P300 latency became significant about 17 years later at the age of around 54 years. The effect of age on P300 in DS was due to the prolonged P300 latency in the 16 individuals who showed signs of dementia.

Confirmation that increases in P300 latency reflect the development of dementia in adults with DS was provided in another study by the same group of researchers (Muir et al. 1988). A total of 65 individuals with DS were followed up and retested 2 years after the initial recordings were undertaken by Blackwood et al. (1988). The number of individuals who showed clinical evidence of dementia had increased by a further 14%. Of those subjects who showed clinical deterioration over a period of 2 years, 75% exhibited an increase in P300 latency. None of the fragile X syndrome group when retested showed a significant change after 2 years. The authors concluded that latency of the auditory evoked potential is a useful test for dementia in adults with DS. However, no studies have replicated these findings since the original work was reported, and in the original studies no information was provided about compliance with testing and how many individuals were excluded prior to involvement in the study.

Visual evoked potentials

A number of researchers have previously reported abnormalities in visual evoked potentials (VEPs) in the general population with DAD (Visser et al. 1976; Moore 1997; Coburn et al. 2003). The principal findings are a delay in the main flash (P2) component but a normal pattern reversal P100 potential (P2–P100 latency). For the DS population, Crapper et al. (1975) were the first to report the use of VEPs to diagnose DAD in a person with DS. Five months before his death, a 54-year-old adult with DS and late-stage DAD underwent repeated flash VEP assessments. The authors found that the late component of the VEPs was virtually absent, a finding which they suggested could be used to improve the clinical diagnosis of DAD.

Prasher et al. (1994), as part of their previous longitudinal research, investigated the accuracy of the P2–P100 latency reported in the general population as a measure for clinical DAD in 44 individuals with DS and 40 age- and sex-matched controls from the general population. The mean age of the DS sample was 45.3 years (range 14–71 years). In total, 14 subjects (64%) were over the age of 40 years, when virtually all individuals with DS show neuropathological changes of AD (Mann 1988). Eight individuals were diagnosed as showing clinical changes of DAD according to modified *DSM-III-R* criteria. Of the 17 people without a diagnosis of DAD, 12 individuals had VEP recordings within normal control limits, one person aged 32 years had an ill-defined P2 but normal P100 result, and four individuals did not cooperate with the procedure. Of the eight people who were diagnosed as suffering from DAD, one had VEP recordings within normal limits, one was unable to cooperate with the procedure and six had abnormal latencies. However, none of these six individuals showed the characteristic P2–

P100 latency changes of DAD found in the general population. Prasher *et al.* (1994) concluded that the use of VEPs to diagnose DAD in adults with DS is limited.

Politoff *et al.* (1996) compared the resting and flash-stimulated EEGs of non-demented adults with DS and age-matched control subjects. In the stimulated EEG, the authors found several cognition-related abnormalities, such as decreased responses to 12-Hz stimulation and disturbance of beta- and gamma-band responses, indicative of decreased responsiveness to photic stimulation, as seen in adults from the general population with DAD. The authors concluded that non-demented individuals with DS and adults with DAD from the general population share several cognition-related EEG abnormalities which are probably due to AD neuropathology.

Electroencephalography in its different forms has a limited role in the assessment or diagnosis of DAD in adults with DS. Standard EEG and evoked potential (auditory or visual) assessments have not been established as reliable tests for DAD either in the general population or in the DS population. These neurophysiological procedures require further research scrutiny with a view to increasing their sensitivity and specificity.

Neuroimaging assessments

Neuroimaging is an important investigatory tool that is used as part of the dementia work-up. It can exclude structural brain lesions which can present with cognitive decline (e.g. tumours, blood clot), and can help to clarify what type of dementia is present (e.g. Alzheimer's disease, vascular dementia). Several types of brain-imaging techniques are now available, but access will depend on local service availability. MRI and CT scans are termed 'structural scans' and show the anatomy of the brain, whereas SPECT and PET scans are termed 'functional scans' and measure brain function.

Computed tomography (CT)

CT is a widely used test in the assessment of DAD because it is readily available and enables the exclusion of other disorders that can cause dementia (e.g. subdural haematoma, brain tumour, hydrocephalus). The role of CT scanning in detecting structural brain changes associated with DAD in the general population has been well documented (Burns *et al.* 1991; Burns and Pearlson 1994; Rossi *et al.* 2004). In general, an association between DAD and cortical atrophy, medial temporal lobe atrophy and ventricular dilatation is seen on CT imaging. The diagnostic value of CT scanning is limited due to marked variability in brain changes associated with normal ageing, an absence of baseline measures in individuals, and the fact that a number of neuropsychiatric diseases present with similar CT abnormalities.

Limited research correlating CT findings with dementia is available for the ID population. Dalton and Crapper (1977) reported CT findings in a study that compared 18 non-demented individuals with DS (age range 19–58 years) with 10 ID controls. The CT findings demonstrated diffuse degeneration in two out of five non-demented individuals with DS, but in both individuals with DS who had dementia. Cerebral atrophy and ventricular enlargement in the latter two cases correlated with profound deterioration in performance measures. Pearlson *et al.* (1990) compared the CT scans of 18 adults with DS (age range 26–70 years), of whom 7 individuals satisfied the criteria for dementia, with 175 healthy controls for evidence of cortical/subcortical atrophy. Cortical atrophy and lateral ventricle dilatation on CT scans correlated with the severity of cognitive impairment. The authors argued that dementia status could be predicted with an accuracy of more than 75% by CT scanning. Schapiro *et al.* (1992) investigated changes on CT scanning in 29 DS subjects and found that there were significant increases in the mean cerebrospinal fluid (CSF) volume and in the mean third ventricle volume in demented older adults with DS compared with younger DS individuals and non-demented older subjects. A number of researchers have shown that the temporal horns are particularly affected (LeMay and Alvarez 1990; Lawlor *et al.* 2001). Enlargement of the suprasellar cistern has been reported to be an early sign of DAD in adults with DS (Maruyama *et al.* 1995), but confirmation of this finding is needed.

Overall, findings from CT studies for DAD in both the non-ID and DS population would suggest that this form of neuroimaging is of value in excluding other causes of dementia, but that as a diagnostic test it has limited sensitivity and specificity. CT changes of DAD may not necessarily change significantly over time, although a person with DS and DAD may deteriorate clinically (Ikeda and Arai 2002). Cortical atrophy and increases in CSF and ventricular volumes are seen in individuals with DAD, but these changes are also found in a large number of non-demented individuals. The difficulties are further increased by the limited resolution of CT scanning and the susceptibility of such scanning to bone artefact.

Single photon emission computed tomography (SPECT)

Measurements of regional cerebral blood flow by SPECT may help to differentiate between DAD and other causes of intellectual decline. Characteristic findings reported in adults in the general population who have DAD are a decrease in regional cerebral blood flow with preservation of arteriovenous differences. Changes are seen in the fronto-temporal region (Tyrrell *et al.* 1990; Matsuda 2001; Dougall *et al.* 2004).

A limited number of studies have investigated changes in SPECT scans in adults with DS (Rae-Grant *et al.* 1991; Puri *et al.* 1994; Jones *et al.* 1997). Melamed *et al.* (1987) measured regional cerebral blood flow (using xenon[133] inhalation) in 14 non-demented individuals with DS (mean age 29 years; age range 16–44 years), in 46 adults from the general population with DAD and in 114 age-matched controls from the general population. Regional cerebral blood flow was reduced in all but one individual with DS compared with age-matched controls. In the 6 individuals with DS who were over 30 years of age, regional cerebral blood flow was reduced slightly (but not significantly) more than in the 8 individuals below this age. The extent of the decreases in regional cerebral blood flow did not differ significantly between different regions of the brain. As none of the individuals with DS had a diagnosis of DAD, the effects of dementia on the SPECT findings could not be determined.

The accuracy and specificity of SPECT scanning in diagnosing dementia in adults with DS was investigated by Deb *et al.* (1992). These researchers performed SPECT scans on 20 adults with DS, four of whom had clinical dementia (diagnosed by a battery of neuropsychological tests, psychiatric interview, physical examination and case-note review). All of the individuals with DS and dementia showed characteristic changes of reduced bilateral perfusion. However, a further 7 individuals (64%) with dementia who had no clinically detectable dementia also showed these changes. The authors concluded that SPECT could not be used as a reliable test for DAD in adults with DS.

Kao *et al.* (1993) found support for the conclusions of Deb *et al.* (1992) when they investigated cerebral blood flow in 14 patients with DS (age range 8–30 years) using SPECT scanning. The scans in all 14 patients invariably showed significant unilateral perfusion defects in the temporal–parietal–occipital region, occasionally combined with small perfusion defects over other discrete cerebral areas. The pattern of regional cerebral blood flow was similar to that in individuals with DAD in the general population, although the DS individuals in the study did not show evidence of DAD.

With regard to diagnosis of DAD, at present the diagnostic accuracy of changes in cerebral blood flow as measured by SPECT scanning is limited. Although SPECT scanning is generally available for functional imaging and it provides different types of information to CT scanning, like CT scanning it has limitations. In particular, changes of hypoperfusion can be seen in both demented and non-demented individuals and may reflect changes associated with the underlying ID or with ageing, rather than with a neurodegenerative disease process.

Positron emission tomography (PET)

PET is a technique that allows quantitative assessment of the rate of glucose utilisation, oxygen consumption and regional cerebral blood flow in the brain. Most individuals in the general population with DAD show regional cerebral hypometabolism compared with age-matched healthy controls. Significant deficits are most commonly seen in the parieto-temporal region and frontal association cortices, but with less apparent changes in the motor cortex, cerebellum and visual cortices (Burns *et al.* 1989; Mielke and Heiss 1998; Poulin and Zakzanis 2002).

As with other neuroimaging investigations in adults with ID, a limited number of studies have investigated PET changes in adults with ID and dementia (Schapiro *et al.* 1987, 1988, 1992; Johanson *et al.* 1991; Azari *et al.* 1994). Schapiro *et al.* (1987) studied the cerebral metabolism of radioactive glucose in 14 healthy adults with DS (age range 19–33 years), in four healthy adults with DS aged over 35 years, and in two adults with DS with modified *DSM-III* criteria (American Psychiatric Association 1987) for the diagnosis of dementia. These findings were compared with the rate of cerebral metabolism of glucose in 15 healthy men aged 20–35 years and 20 healthy men aged 45–64 years. The authors found that the mean rate of hemispheric cerebral metabolism of glucose in the older DS group was significantly (23%) lower than that in the younger DS group. Statistically significant decreases in regional glucose metabolism were also present in all lobar regions. The two older demented DS individuals had the lowest and the third lowest figures for glucose utilisation. The person with the second lowest value developed dementia within one year of her test result. The mean rate of hemispheric cerebral metabolism of glucose has been reported to be 28% lower in DS adults with DAD (Schapiro *et al.* 1988). Marked hypometabolism was evident in the parietal and temporal lobes.

Horwitz *et al.* (1990) correlated cerebral metabolic rates determined by PET scanning with [^{18}F]-2-fluoro-2-deoxy-D-glucose for 14 young healthy adults with DS (aged under 34 years) with those for 24 age-matched healthy controls from the general population. The regional-to-global ratios of resting glucose utilisation were compared for the two groups, and the authors found that the DS group had smaller correlations for region pairs within and between the frontal and parietal lobes. The authors concluded that there was functional disruption of neural circuits in the brains of individuals with DS even prior to the onset of clinical DAD.

Azari *et al.* (1994) specifically investigated frontal-parietal glucose uptake function in adults with DS and dementia (*n* = 4; mean age 56.0 years), compared with that in adults with DS but without clinical dementia (*n* = 10; mean age 47.2 years). These researchers found that the adults with DS and dementia showed the same pattern of frontal-parietal glucose metabolism as was seen in demented adults from the general population. Three years later the same researchers reported findings for 12 adults with DS who had undergone at least three cognitive and PET evaluations over a period of 8–12 years (Pietrini *et al.* 1997). For those individuals who remained well over this period no significant decline in cerebral glucose metabolism was seen. However, for the two individuals who developed dementia a sharp decline in metabolism in the temporo-parietal region was observed.

It has been proposed that temporal cortex hypermetabolism may occur in adults with DS prior to the onset of dementia (Haier *et al.* 2003). These authors postulated that inferior temporal/entorhinal cortex hypermetabolism may reflect a compensatory response early in DAD progression. Compensatory responses may subsequently fail, leading to neurodegenerative processes that present at a later date as glucose hypometabolism accompanied by clinical signs of dementia.

The validity of PET as an accurate test for diagnosing DAD remains uncertain. Its role in the assessment of DAD in adults with ID has yet to be established. Although PET scanning can demonstrate age-related change in adults with DS (Cutler 1986), and may demonstrate some of the typical changes of DAD in the DS population as seen in adults from the general population with dementia, its role is limited by methodological issues similar to those for CT and SPECT scanning. In particular these include inappropriate controls, limited sensitivity and specificity, and a lack of studies correlating findings with post-mortem data.

Magnetic resonance imaging (MRI)

MRI is now a readily available form of investigation. However, not everyone can comply with the procedure, which in up to 20% of individuals can be quite claustrophobic (*see* 10, colour plate section). MRI displays the demarcation of grey and white matter of the brain more clearly than many other neuroimaging techniques. It is extremely useful in studies of intracranial disorders such as cerebral tumours, cerebrovascular events and demyelinating disorders (Besson 1994). Compared with CT, MRI has superior soft-tissue contrast resolution, multiplanar imaging capability, no biological hazards associated with its use, and less risk of artefact in the images (*see* Figures 6.1a and b).

MRI is based on the fact that the commonest nucleus in the body is the hydrogen nucleus (proton). Protons usually spin randomly, but when placed in a

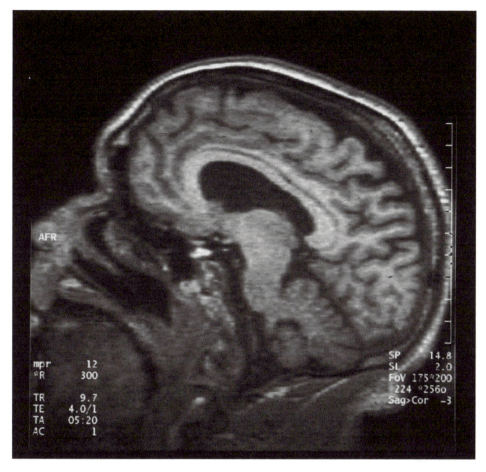

Figure 6.1a Normal MRI scan in elderly person with Down syndrome: sagittal view.

static magnetic field they all align in the same direction. A radio-frequency pulse is administered which transiently alters the direction of the protons. When the pulse is stopped, the protons realign and in doing so release energy that can be detected by sensors, which with the aid of sophisticated computers can convert this energy into images.

The procedure involves the patient lying on a couch with a receiver coil positioned quite closely over the head and upper body. A volumetric brain scan can take 20–30 minutes to complete. Several imaging sequences are undertaken in different planes, each lasting for several minutes. The patient must remain completely still, as movement impairs the quality of the images. Claustrophobia is a significant problem, and occasionally general anaesthesia may be required. Over-sedation is a serious concern in patients with ID (Prasher *et al.* 2003b).

During the last decade a number of studies have been reported that have investigated the role of MRI in detecting anatomical and structural changes in adults with DAD in the general population (*see* Table 6.2). The majority of these studies have demonstrated varying degrees of general cortical atrophy, focal atrophy (particularly in the hippocampal formation and temporal lobes) and

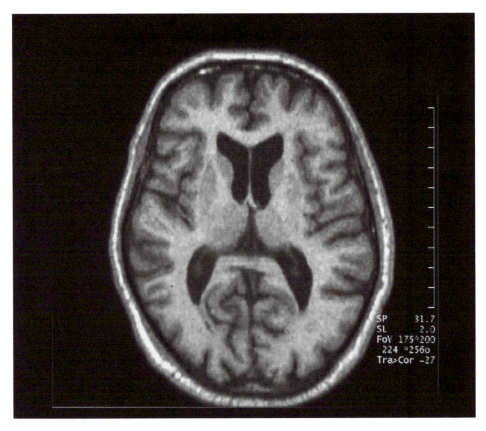

Figure 6.1b Normal MRI scan in elderly person with Down syndrome: horizontal view.

white-matter hyperintensities. The latter are non-specific and are seen in normal ageing and in dementias other than DAD.

A limited number of studies have been published investigating MRI changes in adults with DS (*see* Table 6.3), but few of them have compared findings for DS adults with and without DAD.

One of the earliest studies was by Pelz *et al.* (1986), who found no significant lesions on MRI scanning in seven non-demented adults with DS (age range 17–45 years). However, age-related atrophy without significant white-matter abnormalities was seen in three adults aged 25, 26 and 45 years, respectively. Weis *et al.* (1991) investigated volumetric MRI findings in seven non-demented adults with DS (mean age 38 years; age range 30–45 years) and in seven healthy controls from the general population (mean age 38 years; age range 36–44 years). The mean whole brain volume and the cerebral cortex and cerebellum volumes were significantly smaller on absolute measurements for the DS group compared with the control group. The ventricles were not significantly larger in the DS group. After normalisation of structures for the whole brain volume, none of the structures showed a significant difference.

Kesslak *et al.* (1994) reported a significantly larger parahippocampal gyrus and smaller hippocampus, frontal cortex and cerebellum in 13 individuals with DS (age range 23–51 years) compared with 13 age-matched controls from the general

Table 6.2 Studies investigating MRI changes in the DS population

Studies	Number of DS subjects	Age (years)	Findings
Pelz et al. (1986)	7	Age range 17–45	No significant abnormalities in healthy adults. Age-related atrophy found in three individuals
Weis et al. (1991)	7	Mean age 38.0	Non-demented individuals. After normalisation no differences compared with controls
Kesslak et al. (1994)	13	Age range 23–51	Larger parahippocampal and smaller hippocampus, frontal cortex and cerebellum volumes for DS group compared with controls. Atrophic changes seen in two demented individuals
Raz et al. (1995)	13	Mean age 35.2	Non-demented individuals. No relationship between total brain size and level of intelligence
Roth et al. (1996)	30	Mean age 39.0	Hypointensity of basal ganglia, white-matter changes, atrophy more marked in demented cases
Frangou et al. (1997)	17	Mean age 39.2	Superior temporal gyrus and volume beneath planum temporale smaller in DS individuals than in controls
Aylward et al. (1997)	32	Mean age 40.3	No significant differences between demented and non-demented individuals
Pearlson et al. (1998)	50	66.0	Generalised atrophy, third ventricular enlargement and reduction in total brain volume in demented individuals
Prasher et al. (2003b)	38	Age range 26–78	Reduction in total brain, temporal lobe and hippocampal volumes and increased ventricular volume in demented individuals.

This table is based on the original that appeared as Table 1, p. 92 in Prasher V, Cumella S, Natarajan K, Rolfe E, Shah S and Haque S (2003b) Magnetic resonance imaging, Down's syndrome and Alzheimer's disease: research and clinical implications. *J Intellect Disabil Res.* **47**: 90–100.

population. In individuals with DS there was a significant increase in ventricular area with age, and a significant age-related decrease in hippocampal area. In two individuals with DS and dementia, atrophic changes of the hippocampus and parahippocampal gyrus were observed, and enlarged ventricles similar to those seen in adults in the general population with DAD were seen.

Roth et al. (1996) retrospectively reviewed MRI scans of 30 adults with DS and 30 age- and sex-matched controls from the general population. Ten of the individuals with DS were diagnosed as having clinical dementia. Scans were evaluated for evidence of atrophy, white-matter lesions and hypointensity of the basal ganglia. In the DS group all but one individual had at least one abnormal marker on their MRI scan. The most commonly reported abnormality was

Table 6.3 Studies investigating MRI changes in DAD in the general population

Studies	Number of AD subjects	Mean age (years)	Findings
Kertesz et al. (1990)	27	73.3	Increased white-matter changes
McDonald et al. (1991)	22	64.1	Increased periventricular hyperintensities, ventriculomegaly and sulcal widening
Jernigan et al. (1991)	25	70.0	Significant loss in all cortical and subcortical regions. No significant reduction in white-matter volume
Killiany et al. (1993)	8	72.0	Reduction in hippocampus and temporal lobes. Increase in volume of lateral ventricles
Erkinjuntti et al. (1993)	34	70.0	Temporal lobe atrophy
Cuenod et al. (1993)	11	77.4	Atrophy of amygdala
DeCarli et al. (1995)	31	68.1	Reduction in frontal and temporal lobe volumes
Laakso et al. (1995)	32	66.0	Smaller hippocampal and left frontal lobe volumes
O'Brien et al. (1996)	61	71.2	White-matter changes adjacent to ventricular system. Hippocampal atrophy
Pitkanen et al. (1996)	55	69.9	Atrophy of hippocampus
Lehtovirta et al. (1996)	58	69.9	Atrophy of hippocampus, amygdala and medial temporal lobe
Pantel et al. (1997)	20	75.6	Reduction in whole brain volume and in volumes of frontal and temporal lobes and amygdala–hippocampus complex
Cahn et al. (1998)	20	71.7	Differential atrophy of hippocampus and temporal lobe and lateral ventricle dilatation with cognitive deficits
Harvey et al. (1999)	11	78.8	Atrophy of left temporal lobe and parahippocampal gyri

hypointensity of the basal ganglia, followed by white-matter changes, and the least often reported abnormality was generalised atrophy. Abnormalities were more severe in demented than in non-demented individuals with DS.

Aylward et al. (1997) determined the effects of age and neuropsychological status on the volume of the basal ganglia in 32 adults with DS. Five subjects were diagnosed clinically as having dementia. The authors found that the total brain volume and total brain volume plus CSF volume were significantly smaller for the non-demented DS group than for general population controls. Measurements of the basal ganglia volumes indicated that individuals with DS had significantly larger putamen volumes than control subjects, but did not differ in total basal ganglia, caudate and globus pallidus volumes. In the DS group, age was negatively correlated with volumes of putamen and total basal ganglia, and with total brain volume. No significant difference was found for basal ganglia or brain volumes when demented and non-demented individuals with DS were compared.

Pearlson *et al.* (1998) investigated MRI evidence of brain changes in 50 individuals with DS (with and without dementia) and compared their findings with those for 23 controls from the general population. A clinical diagnosis of dementia was made for 11 individuals with DS (who were statistically significantly older than the non-demented DS group). The DS group had a non-significant tendency to have a smaller hippocampus, significantly larger lateral ventricles and a higher frequency of posterior fossa arachnoid cysts/megacisterna magna, and fewer scans were rated as normal. Quantitatively, total brain, grey matter, left hippocampus and amygdala volumes were reduced in the DS group. Comparison of scans from DS individuals with and without dementia showed that the former had more generalised atrophy, mesial temporal shrinkage, third ventricular enlargement, and reduced total brain, left hippocampus and left amydala volumes.

Prasher *et al.* (2003b) investigated the role of MRI in detecting structural brain changes specifically associated with DAD in 38 adults with DS, with or without dementia. The findings of the study suggested that standard two-dimensional MRI scans did not reliably demonstrate changes associated with DAD in adults with DS. For volumetric results (controlling for differences in total brain volume),

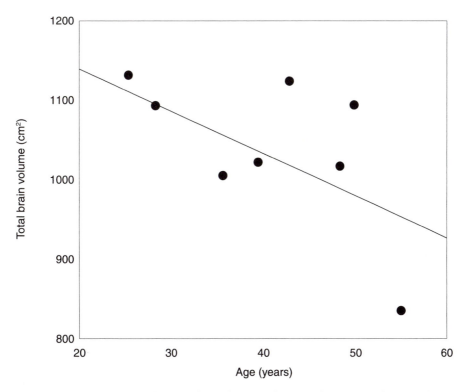

Figure 6.2 Age-related total brain volume for non-demented Down syndrome subjects.

none of the differences in findings between DAD and non-DAD individuals in the study were statistically significant at the 5% significance level. A trend towards a reduction in total brain volume and in temporal lobe and hippocampal volumes and an increase in the ventricular volume was seen. A significant age-related reduction in total brain volume was found (*see* Figure 6.2). The findings were consistent with those reported for adults in the general population with DAD.

As was mentioned earlier, poor compliance of DS individuals with MRI testing and post-procedure complications are major concerns and significant factors limiting the use of MRI in older adults with ID (Prasher *et al.* 2003b). The authors found that a significant number of individuals with DS did not cooperate with the investigation, even after being given sedation. In that study, only 11 of 19 individuals with DS and DAD had MRI scans of a satisfactory quality. Over-sedation was a serious concern, and the authors commented that without the appropriate medical support, death of an adult with DS could result.

Overall, the MRI findings suggest that the cerebrum and cerebellum volumes for adults with DS are small, but they are not disproportionately reduced in relation to

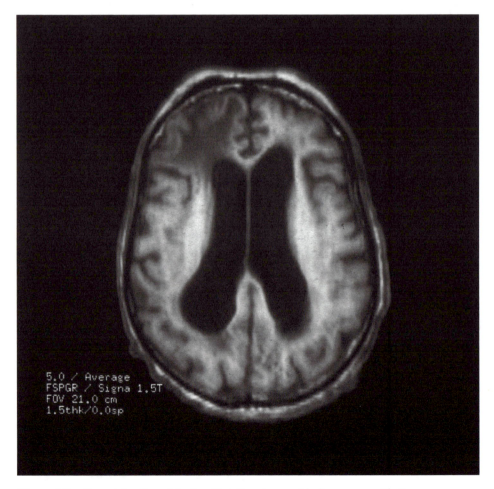

Figure 6.3a Gross lateral ventricular dilatation in an elderly person with Down syndrome and dementia in Alzheimer's disease (horizontal view).

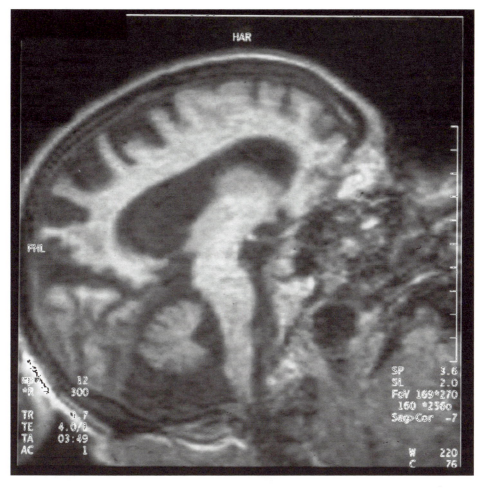

Figure 6.3b Marked brain atrophy and gross lateral ventricular dilatation in an elderly person with Down syndrome and dementia in Alzheimer's disease.

the total brain volume. The volume of the basal ganglia is also not disproportionately reduced, but the parahippocampal gyrus may be enlarged. Age-related abnormalities (e.g. reduction in total brain volume and increase in ventricular volume) are present. Such abnormalities are most marked in individuals with DS and severe DAD (*see* Figure 6.3a and 6.3b). At present MRI has a limited role in the routine assessment and diagnosis of DAD in adults with DS.

Summary

The diagnosis of DAD in adults in the general population can sometimes be difficult, but it is even more problematic in older adults with ID. There must be a characteristic decline in a person's level of intellectual and social functioning, together with changes in personality, emotions and behaviour. For adults with ID, clinical deterioration associated with DAD may be detected by neuropsychological measures. However, the reliability and validity of such measures remain questionable. They may be appropriate to a strongly biased and highly selective sample, but studies demonstrating their applicability to the ID population as a whole are still needed.

A number of research studies have investigated the potential of neurophysiological and neuroimaging measures for diagnosing DAD in all individuals irrespective of their underlying level of intelligence. These have ranged from inexpensive and readily available tests (e.g. electroencephalography) to more expensive and limited-access assessments (e.g. PET scans). Research studies of older adults with ID have involved limited numbers of individuals with DS, and few with DAD. Neuroimaging investigations at present have a limited role in the field of ID. There are few normative data for ageing adults with ID, and furthermore the risks involved in neuroimaging procedures have not been fully evaluated.

Chapter 7

Management and treatment of dementia

Introduction

The management and treatment of dementia in Alzheimer's disease (DAD) in people with intellectual disability (ID) remains an area of considerable interest, but surprisingly few good-quality research data are available with regard to appropriate forms of management. To fill this gap, an international working group under the auspices of American Association on Mental Retardation–International Association for the Scientific Study of Intellectual Disabilities (AAMR-IASSID) published practice guidelines to aid clinical practice and highlight further areas of research (Janicki *et al.* 1996). This chapter will principally focus on drug treatments. However, it is important that drug treatment remains only one form of management of dementia, and indeed it may not be the best form of treatment, as other approaches such as carer support, changes in the environment and behavioural therapy may be more appropriate. Although it is important to treat the underlying illness, it is equally important to provide care for the person as a whole. The management of a particular problem, such as aggression, may be amenable to treatment with antipsychotic medication, but other issues such as carer stress, and risk to the individual and to others also need to be assessed and managed.

Drugs are commonly prescribed for dementia, both in the general population and in people with ID, and can be prescribed for up to 70–75% of individuals living in residential or nursing homes. Concern has been expressed in the general population about the overuse and high rates of prescribing of antipsychotic medication to treat dementia in facilities where medication may not be reviewed on a regular basis, marked side-effects are evident, and the specific reason for initiating treatment is unknown.

A reduction in the use of medication and greater use of non-drug therapies in residential homes is important. Greater emphasis should be given to staff engaging people with dementia in activities and occupations that can maintain their skills, and to keeping individuals active. However, due to staff shortages and low morale, it is not uncommon for staff themselves to initiate the use of medication. Indiscriminate use of medication is therefore an important area that needs to be further assessed and monitored. Once the clinical diagnosis of DAD has been made, a treatment plan must be formulated. This plan should include the use of anti-dementia therapy along with psychological intervention to temporarily improve the disease process or slow the rate of decline.

Drug treatments for DAD

Prior to initiating drug treatments for dementia, a detailed assessment of the patient should be undertaken, in particular to rule out any underlying physical disorder that might be causing the presenting problem (*see* Chapter 5). It is not uncommon for a physical illness, particularly if it is associated with pain, to present as behavioural problems, especially in elderly people who may have limited communication and sensory skills. As part of the assessment, it is important to establish exactly why medication is being prescribed, and how it is likely to be beneficial. Any alternative interventions that could be tried prior to the use of medication should be discussed with carers. These may include practical support, and increased support from voluntary agencies.

Current medication, particularly psychotropic drugs (which may include antipsychotics, tranquillisers and antidepressants), should be reviewed. Such medication may need to be altered prior to the initiation of new treatment. It cannot be overemphasised that initiation of any treatment must be safe and not harmful to the patient. Elderly people with ID may have low body weight, be generally quite frail and have ongoing physical illnesses, which can be significantly worsened by the use of medication (e.g. sedatives leading to an increase in falls).

An assessment is needed of whether the person will take medication, and also in what form it would be most appropriately administered if taken. Some people with deterioration of dementia may be unable to swallow tablets, or indeed may find it impossible to take any form of medication at all due to associated swallowing difficulties. The method of administration and the times of day at which medication should be given need to be discussed with the appropriate carers. Certainly there are ethical issues regarding the treatment of people who may not give consent to treatment. This issue is beyond the remit of this book, but does need to be discussed with carers and family members. Treatment may be necessary within the framework of mental health legislation.

As should be the practice for people with ID, but is even more important for older adults with ID who may develop dementia, any medication should be initiated at a low dose and the dose increased gradually. It is usually necessary to give lower doses than those used in younger people. This is because of impaired drug absorption in older adults with ID, alterations in the drug action, and the increased risk of drug interactions. Such differences can alter blood levels and the bioavailability of the drug. It may be advisable to initiate treatment for a trial period and review it frequently in order to ascertain whether it has any benefit, and in particular to monitor any side-effects. If any medication is discontinued it is best to reduce the dose gradually. The benefits, side-effects and interactions of medications should be discussed with carers and, where appropriate, written information employing user-friendly language should be provided. This is particularly important in the case of the newer drugs, which have yet to be widely used in people with ID.

Drug treatment for DAD falls into three main areas. First, it aims to improve cognitive function in older adults with DAD by treating the underlying cause of AD. Secondly, drug treatment is used to treat psychological and behavioural symptoms and signs that are associated with the dementia. Thirdly, the treatment involves the management of coexisting physical health problems associated with dementia (e.g. urinary tract infections, chest infections).

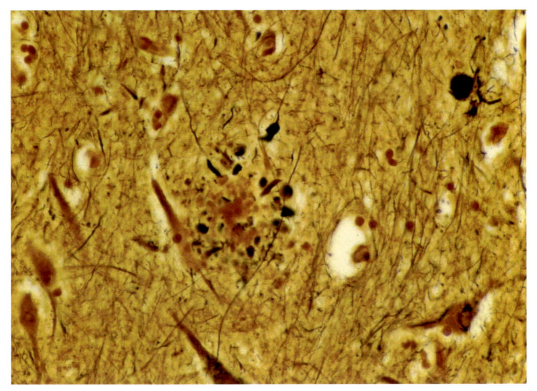

1 Typical senile plaque seen in Alzheimer's disease.

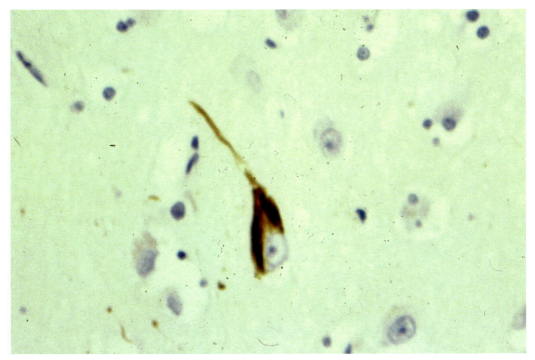

2 Neurofibrillary tangle seen in Alzheimer's disease.

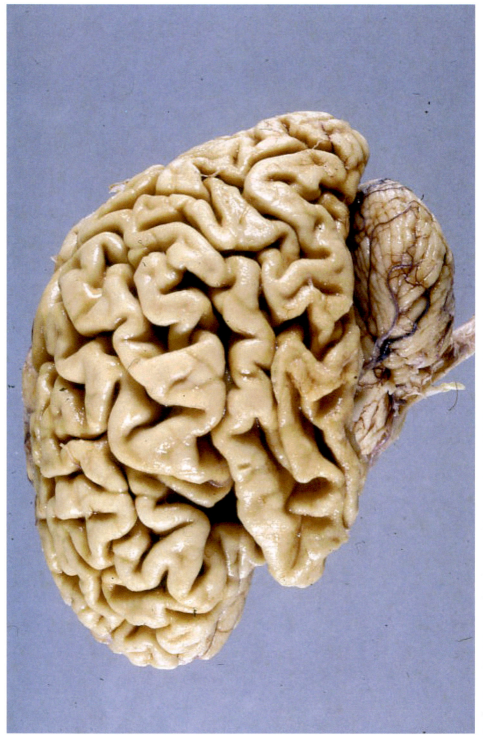

3 Generalised cerebral atrophy seen in Alzheimer's disease.

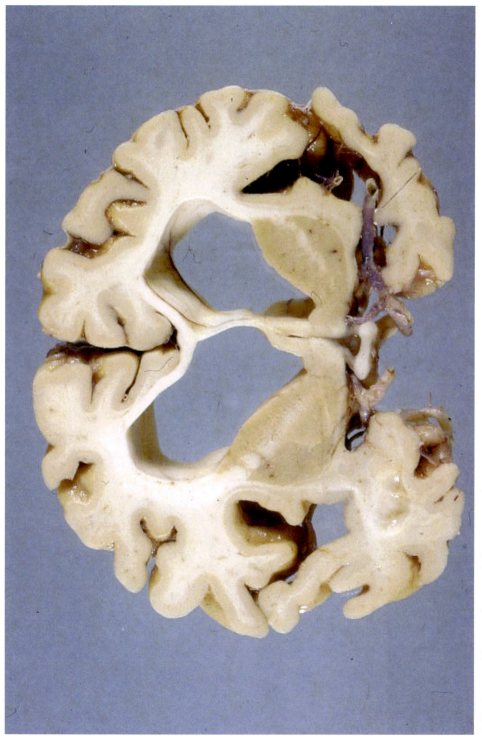

4 Enlarged lateral ventricles seen in Alzheimer's disease.

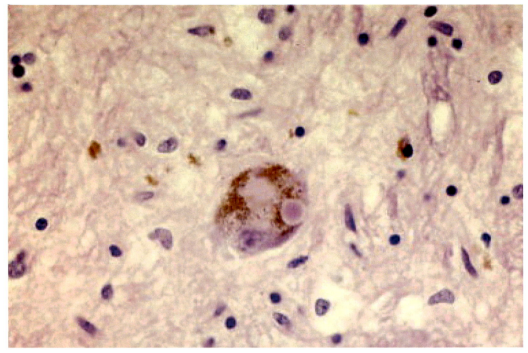

5 Lewy body seen in Lewy body dementia.

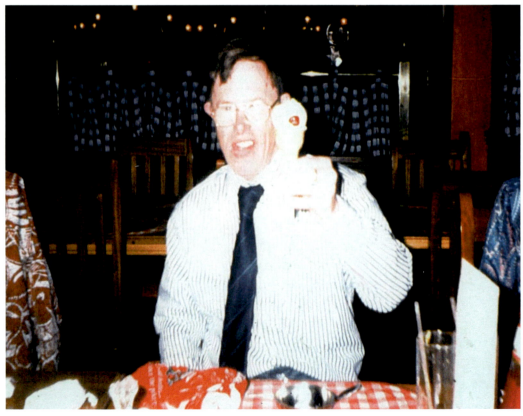

6 J aged 49 years, fit and well.

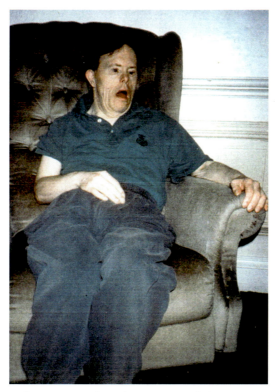

7 J 5 years after the onset of dementia, now resident in a nursing home.

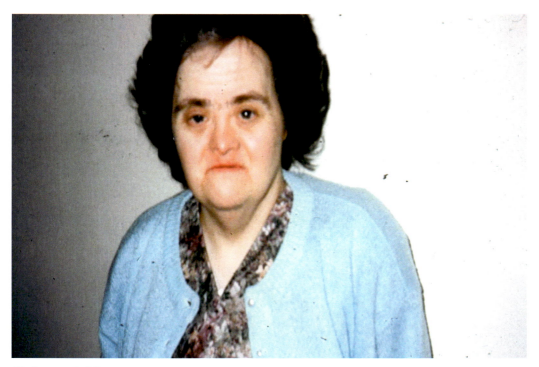

8 A aged 46 years.

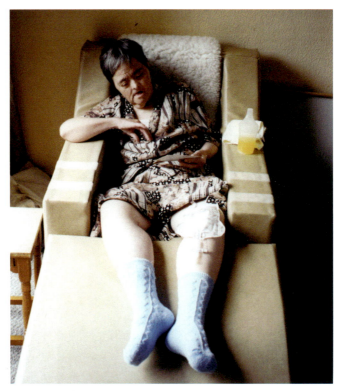

9 A aged 55 years, with severe dementia.

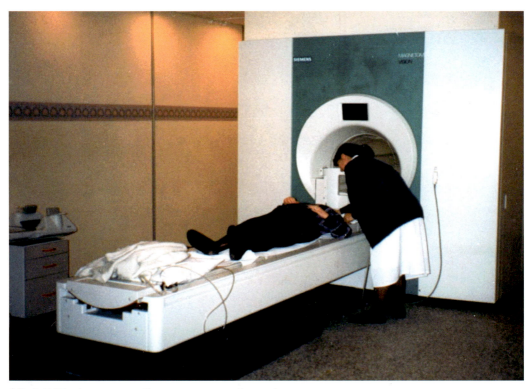

10 1.5 Tesla magnetic resonance imaging scanner.

Specific anti-dementia drug therapy

The development of the most recent anti-dementia drugs is based on the current *cholinergic hypothesis* with regard to Alzheimer's disease (Farlow 2002). There is strong evidence that there is a reduction in the activity of acetylcholine within the brain due to the loss of cholinergic neurons in the nucleus basilis of Meynert, and loss of projections to the hippocampus and mesio-temporal regions of the brain (Poirier *et al.* 1999). The reduction in cholinergic activity is thought to lead to a decline in cognition function and to related behavioural symptoms. Historically, researchers have tried to improve acetylcholine function within the brain by a number of mechanisms (*see* Table 7.1).

An alternative to the cholinergic hypothesis for AD is the hypothesis that glutamate-mediated neurotoxicity is involved in the pathogenesis of AD and this is the principal abnormality (Danysz *et al.* 2000). According to this hypothesis, glutamate receptors (N-methyl-D-aspartate; NMDA) are overactive, leading to impairment of β-amyloid and/or tau protein metabolism, which results in neuropathological changes of AD. Memantine is the only licensed anti-dementia drug that acts on glutamate receptors.

The most commonly used form of anti-dementia drug treatment involves reducing degeneration of acetylcholine by cholinesterase inhibitors. Tacrine was the first tested and clinically prescribed cholinesterase inhibitor. However, due to its hepatotoxicity it is no longer available for clinical use. More recently, considerable evidence has been found that the cholinesterase inhibitors donepezil, rivastigmine and galantamine are effective in slowing down the rate of degeneration associated with DAD in the general population (Dooley and Lamb 2000; Van Den Berg *et al.* 2000; Ballard 2002). Tables 7.2 and 7.3 list details of the pharmacological and pharmacokinetic differences between the various anti-dementia drugs.

Mohs *et al.* (2001) reported a study of 431 people with DAD in the general population who were randomised to either donepezil 10 mg or placebo. The authors found that the former group maintained their clinical skills for 72% longer, and were less likely to decline (by approximately 40%) over the year compared with the placebo group. Overall, a number of studies demonstrated a benefit in global functioning, cognitive abilities, neuropsychiatric symptoms, behavioural problems, daily living skills and a reduction in carer stress (Burns *et al.* 1999; Wimo *et al.* 2003). In the UK, the National Institute for Clinical

Table 7.1 Mechanism of action of cholinergic anti-dementia drugs

Mechanism of action	Drug
Precursor loading	Choline, lecithin
Stimulation of transmitter release	Linopirodine
Slowing of transmitter degeneration	Tacrine
Cholinesterase inhibition	Donepezil, rivastigmine, galantamine, metrifonate
Direct selective agonist activity	Xanomeline, milameline

Table 7.2 Summary of pharmacological parameters of anti-dementia drugs

Drug	Chemical class	Action	Type of inhibition	Route of administration	Frequency of administration	Given with food?	Dosage/day	Indications
Donepezil	Piperidine	AChE inhibitor	Rapidly reversible	Oral – tablets	Once a day	No	5–10 mg	Mild to moderate AD
Rivastigmine	Carbamate	AChE and BChE inhibitor	Pseudo-reversible	Oral – capsules and solution	Twice a day	Yes	6–12 mg	Mild to moderate AD
Galantamine	Phenanthrene alkaloid	AChE inhibitor	Rapidly reversible	Oral – tablets	Twice a day	Yes	16–24 mg	Mild to moderately severe AD
Memantine	Glutamatergic modulator	NMDA antagonist	–	Oral – tablets and solution	Twice a day	No	10–20 mg	Moderately severe to severe AD

This table is based on the original that appeared as Table 1, p. 510 in Prasher VP (2004) Review of donepezil, rivastigmine, galanatamine and memantine for the treatment of dementia in AD in adults with Down syndrome: implications for the intellectual disability population. *Int J Geriatr Psychiatry.* **19**: 1–7.

Table 7.3 Summary of pharmacokinetic parameters of anti-dementia drugs

Drug	Time to reach maximum concentration (hours)	Elimination half-life (hours)	Protein binding (%)	Total body clearance* (L/hour/kg)	Time to steady state (days)	Excretion
Donepezil	3–5	50–70	96	0.13	14–22	Hepatic
Rivastigmine	0.5–2.0	0.6–2.0	43	N/A		Hepatic
Galantamine	1.2	5–7	<20	N/A	2	Hepatic and renal
Memantine	3–8	60–100	45	N/A	11	Renal

*Drug clearance from plasma.

This table is based on the original that appeared as Table 2, p. 511 in Prasher VP (2004) Review of donepezil, rivastigmine, galanatamine and memantine for the treatment of dementia in AD in adults with Down syndrome: implications for the intellectual disability population. *Int J Geriatr Psychiatry.* **19**: 1–7.

Excellence (2001) and in the USA the American Academy of Neurology (Doody *et al.* 2001) concluded that anti-dementia drugs have a significant benefit in patients with DAD, and that these agents should be made available.

Each anti-dementia drug should be started at a sub-therapeutic dosage and the dose gradually increased. A baseline ECG may be required for some individuals in order to exclude cardiac abnormalities prior to the commencement of therapy. Medication may need to be withdrawn if tolerance or compliance is poor or if the patient's condition continues to deteriorate rapidly. There are a number of medical conditions in which anti-dementia drugs should be used with caution (*see* Table 7.4). These include sick sinus syndrome, supraventricular conduction abnormalities, history of peptic ulcer, chronic airway disease, anaesthesia, and hepatic and renal impairment. All of the anti-dementia drugs discussed above are generally well tolerated, and most of the adverse events that may occur are mild and transient. The commonly reported adverse events are listed in Table 7.5.

Whereas several studies investigating the role of anti-dementia drugs in the general population have been published, few studies (Kishnani *et al.* 1999; Lott *et al.* 2002; Prasher *et al.* 2002b, 2003a, 2005; Margallo-Lana *et al.* 2003) have been reported on the use of drug therapy to treat dementia in adults with DS. Virtually all of the information that is available is on the use of donepezil. Extremely limited information is available on the use of rivastigmine, galantamine and memantine in the ID population (Prasher 2004; Prasher *et al.* 2003a).

Kishnani *et al.* (1999) reported their findings for four adults with DS who were treated with up to 10 mg donepezil for between 26 and 68 weeks. The two younger individuals (aged 24 and 27 years) showed no evidence of dementia, but the two older subjects (aged 38 and 64 years) met the *DSM-IV* criteria for dementia. On the measurement of adaptive behaviour there was an improvement in scores for the non-demented individuals but little change for the demented subjects.

Using more rigid methodological criteria than those employed by Kishnani *et al.* (1999), Prasher *et al.* (2002b) published findings from a 24-week, double-blind placebo-controlled trial of donepezil in 30 patients with DS and DAD. The Dementia Questionnaire for Persons with Mental Retardation (DMR) (Evenhuis *et al.* 1990) was used as the primary outcome measure (global impression), and a

Table 7.4 Conditions in which anti-dementia therapy should be used with caution

Drug	Condition
Donepezil	Sick sinus syndrome, supraventricular conduction abnormalities, history of peptic ulcers, asthma, chronic obstructive airway disease, hepatic impairment
Rivastigmine	Renal impairment, hepatic impairment, sick sinus syndrome, supraventricular conduction abnormalities, history of peptic ulcers, asthma, chronic obstructive airway disease
Galantamine	Sick sinus syndrome, supraventricular conduction abnormalities, history of peptic ulcers, asthma, chronic obstructive airway disease, hepatic impairment, urinary obstruction
Memantine	Renal impairment. Caution in patients with epilepsy or cardiovascular disorders

This table is based on the original that appeared as Table 4, p. 513 in Prasher VP (2004) Review of donepezil, rivastigmine, galanatamine and memantine for the treatment of dementia in AD in adults with Down syndrome: implications for the intellectual disability population. *Int J Geriatr Psychiatry.* 19: 1–7.

Table 7.5 Commonly occurring side-effects of the anti-dementia drugs

Adverse event	Donepezil	Rivastigmine	Galantamine	Memantine
Nausea	+	+	+	
Diarrhoea	+	+	+	+
Insomnia	+	+	+	+
Fatigue	+	+	+	+
Vomiting	+	+	+	+
Muscle cramps	+			
Anorexia	+	+	+	
Headache	+	+	+	+
Dizziness	+	+	+	+
Syncope	+	+	+	
Urinary incontinence	+			
Psychiatric disturbances	+	+	+	+
Rash	+	+	+	
Pruritus	+			
Weight loss		+	+	
Abdominal pain		+		
Drowsiness		+		
Hallucinations				+
Cardiac changes	+		+	+
Cystitis			+	+
Increased libido			+	

This table is based on the original that appeared as Table 3, p. 513 in Prasher VP (2004) Review of donepezil, rivastigmine, galanatamine and memantine for the treatment of dementia in AD in adults with Down syndrome: implications for the intellectual disability population. *Int J Geriatr Psychiatry.* 19: 1–7.

number of other instruments were used to assess secondary outcome measures of cognition, neuropsychiatric features and adaptive behaviour. The donepezil group showed a statistically non-significant reduction in deterioration in global functioning, cognitive skills and adaptive behaviour. No serious medical event occurred during the study period. The authors concluded that donepezil should be used to treat DAD in adults with DS.

Lott *et al.* (2002) investigated the role of donepezil in the treatment of dementia in 9 adults with DS compared with 6 historical control subjects. The treatment period was 83–182 days, with a dosage of up to 10 mg daily. Dementia was assessed before treatment and after an average interval of 5 months using the Down Syndrome Dementia Scale (DSDS) (Gedye 1995). A significant improvement in dementia scores was seen in individuals who were treated with donepezil.

Prasher *et al.* (2003a) went on to report on an open-label study (of duration 104 weeks) that evaluated the long-term safety and efficacy of donepezil in the treatment of DAD in adults with DS. Patients in this open-label study had previously completed the 24-week randomised double-blind placebo-controlled trial (Prasher *et al.* 2002b), and were followed up using the same assessments as in the 24-week study. Individuals who were treated with donepezil in the 24-week study continued with treatment (the 'always on donepezil' [AOD] group). They were compared with those initially on placebo in the 24-week study, who were continued on no active medication in the open-label phase (the 'never on donepezil' [NOD] group). The primary outcome measure was the DMR.

Figure 7.1 shows the change in total DMR scores for the two groups in the open-phase study. For the NOD group there was deterioration over the time

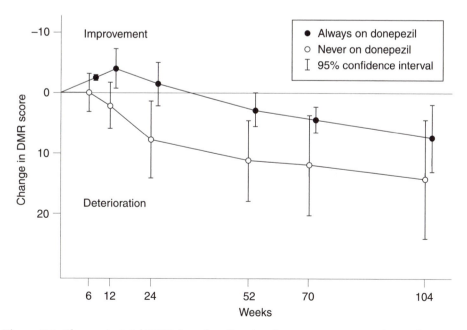

Figure 7.1 Change in total DMR from baseline for the two groups over the study period. Modified from figure 6, p. 135 in Prasher (2003) The role of donepezil in the treatment of dementia in Alzheimer's disease in adults with Down syndrome. In: JA Malard (ed.) *Focus on Down Syndrome Research*. Nova Biomedical Press, New York.

period of the study. For the AOD group there was some improvement in DAD scores, but after approximately 24 weeks there was a gradual deterioration in scores. Over the 104-week period the rate of deterioration in dementia was less for the AOD group than for the NOD group. At 104 weeks the deterioration in global functioning and adaptive behaviour was statistically significantly less for the treated DS individuals with DAD. This study demonstrated that donepezil was beneficial in the treatment of DAD in the DS population for up to 2 years.

Prasher *et al.* (2005) reported their findings with regard to the use of rivastigmine in older adults with DS who had an *ICD-10* (World Health Organization 1992) diagnosis of DAD over a 24-week period. The results for 17 treated adults were compared with the findings for the placebo group in the donepezil study (Prasher *et al.* 2002b). On the global assessment (DMR scores) there was a deterioration in DAD scores for both groups over the 24-week period. The percentage change was less for the rivastigmine group (7.8%) than for the untreated group (10.7%). There was no statistically significant difference in the rate of decline for the two groups at the 5% level. This non-significance may have been due to the small sample size, rather than to rivastigmine being ineffective. The authors commented that further larger studies are required to clarify this matter, but it seems probable that adults with DS and DAD could benefit from treatment with rivastigmine.

There are difficulties in undertaking rigorous drug trials in the ID population, particular concerns being the problem of small sample size, non-blindness of carers and raters, the different inclusion criteria for DAD, the reliability of the outcome measures used and the type of statistical analysis employed. However, from the available information it would appear that individuals with ID and DAD are likely to benefit from the above anti-dementia drugs, or should at least be given a trial period of treatment in order to assess the efficacy of these drugs.

Non-cholinergic anti-dementia drugs

Non-steroidal anti-inflammatory drugs (NSAIDs)

Findings for adults in the general population would suggest that there is an activated inflammatory response during the neuropathological development of AD, with increases in the inflammatory agents interleukin-1β and S-100β (McGeer and McGeer 1998). Non-steroidal anti-inflammatory drugs (e.g. ibuprofen, naproxen, aspirin) suppress these neuro-inflammatory species and may subsequently decrease the production of amyloid-β (1-42), the main component of senile plaques (Imbimbo 2004). Cross-sectional and retrospective clinical epidemiological studies have demonstrated that anti-inflammatory drugs reduce the prevalence and incidence of DAD in the general population (McGeer and McGeer 1996).

There is some evidence that treatment with NSAIDs can prevent or delay the onset of DAD. However, it remains uncertain whether a high or low dosage of medication is most effective. Adverse effects (e.g. gastrointestinal haemorrhage, dyspepsia) are important concerns to be taken into account prior to commencement of NSAID treatment. No reports have been published on the use of NSAIDs to treat DAD in the ID population.

Anti-oxidants

An alternative theory to the cholinergic hypothesis for the development of DAD is that free radicals damage neurons, leading to neuropathology of AD. It is therefore argued that drugs and/or vitamins that act as either free radical scavengers or anti-oxidants can be beneficial in the treatment of DAD. A number of studies have been reported which suggest that the use of these drugs and/or vitamins (e.g. selegiline, vitamin C and/or vitamin E [α-tocopherol]) can slow down the progression of DAD or prevent the onset of DAD in the general population (Sano *et al.* 1997; Martin 2003). With regard to the ID population, at present findings are awaited from an international double-blind randomised controlled drug trial designed to investigate the benefits of vitamin E therapy in preventing ageing and dementia in older adults with DS. The clinical use of anti-oxidants for the treatment of DAD in the ID population cannot be recommended at present.

Ostrogen

Oestrogen increases cerebral blood flow, enhances neurotrophin release, increases cholinergic activity, promotes cell growth and can reduce β-amyloid deposition. Epidemiological studies of post-menopausal women have suggested that oestrogen replacement therapy may reduce the risk of developing DAD or reduce further deterioration in women who already have DAD (Yaffe *et al.* 1998). A dose–response effect (i.e. the longer the oestrogen administration, the greater the benefit) has been reported. For the ID population there is some epidemiological evidence of an association between DAD and oestrogen deficiency (Schupf and Sergievsky 2002). However, further evidence is still required before oestrogen therapy can be used to treat DAD.

Extract of *Ginkgo biloba*

Extract of *Ginkgo biloba* leaves (a herbal medicine) has been prescribed for a number of neurological problems, and although its action is not fully understood, there is some evidence that it may be beneficial in the general population in improving cognitive function associated with ageing, dementia and DAD (Gertz and Kiefer 2004). It is postulated that the benefits of *Ginkgo biloba* extract are exerted through its anti-oxidant or anti-inflammatory actions.

There are ongoing double-blind placebo-controlled studies to fully establish the efficacy of *Ginkgo biloba* extract for the treatment of DAD in the general population. Caution is required in adults with a history of haemorrhage, as *Ginkgo biloba* can reduce platelet function (Sierpina *et al.* 2003). No information is available for adults with ID.

Non-pharmacological treatments for dementia

The non-pharmacological treatment of DAD is complex, and indeed it could be argued that the vast majority of care is already non-pharmacological, being given by carers themselves. Certainly the environment in which a person with ID and dementia is cared for does have a major impact on the course of the disease. For example, an environment that is dehumanising, which devalues the person with dementia and where carers have prejudiced views will have high rates of behavioural and psychological problems and often an associated high level of pharmacological intervention. Where possible, non-pharmacological management techniques should be considered prior to intervention with medication, and can also be used as adjuncts to drug therapy. There are several general principles which, if implemented, can reduce the distress associated with dementia.

1 Increase the amount of time spent by carer(s) with the person with DAD.
2 Structure the day with recreational and social activities.
3 Intervene with behavioural measures to maintain skills and reduce aggression.
4 Use a person-centred approach to tailor interventions to the individual.
5 Make changes to the environment.
6 Compensate for loss of skills by communicating clearly and repeating instructions.
7 Assess the risk of further harm (e.g. falls).
8 Provide carer support.

Several specific psychological interventions administered by healthcare professionals have been developed to help to manage DAD. However, it is generally accepted that psychological interventions at present do not have the rigour of pharmacological double-blind placebo-controlled trials, not only in the general population but also in the population with ID.

Behavioural approaches

A number of behavioural techniques have been used in older adults with dementia in the general population. These have involved either increasing the patient's level of independence and adaptive behaviour or reducing levels of behavioural disturbance. A detailed assessment is always required for any problematic behaviour. For example, a person who is screaming may be doing so as an expression of pain, or as a means of self-stimulation, rather than to 'seek attention'. Excessive noise making such as shouting, screaming or repeatedly calling may be due to under- or over-stimulation. Greater education and support for carers with regard to training and problem-solving techniques, as well as the use of memory aids, can improve the self-care skills of people with dementia.

Older adults with dementia who are given prompting and praise (e.g. to improve their walking or incontinence) have been shown to maintain skills for longer than individuals who have been subject to carer intervention at an early stage. Wandering is a common feature of DAD, and several techniques involving environmental changes (e.g. using masking tape to mark out areas on the floor, putting mirrors on exit doors, painting particular doors a given colour, such as blue for toilet doors) have been used. Increasing aggression in the late afternoon and evening, described as 'sundowning', has been reported. This may be related to changes in the circadian rhythm due to pathological changes in the brain. Whether exposure to bright light in order to restore the circadian rhythm to normal is beneficial remains controversial. Providing support and training to enable staff to implement consistently and over a specified period both verbal and non-verbal behavioural measures is essential if non-pharmacological intervention is to be successful.

Further research is needed to formally confirm the benefits of such interventions.

Certainly increased support for carers to improve their understanding, communication and management of behavioural problems is of value. Non-pharmacological techniques can be used alongside pharmacological techniques, and are part of a complex general plan of assessment and treatment.

Reality orientation

Reality orientation is a well-established form of psychological intervention for dementia in the general population, and has been used for more than half a century. It can involve individuals or groups. The aim of the treatment is to maintain orientation with regard to time, place and self by active participation in discussions of current events or of activities on a given day. The orientating information is then reinforced by the use of music, memory aids and question-and-answer sessions. Spector *et al.* (2000a) undertook a review of orientation therapy for adults with dementia in the general population and found that the overall results significantly supported the beneficial effects of reality orientation on cognitive function, with a limited improvement in behavioural functions. Some researchers have criticised reality orientation therapy, arguing that it is often applied in a mechanical fashion and is not sensitive to the needs of individuals (Bates *et al.* 2004).

Further research is required on the benefits of reality orientation for older adults with ID who have dementia. How applicable is it to individuals who have underlying intellectual impairment and who even when well may not have been orientated with regard to time? Can it be widely used for adults who present with moderate or severe dementia (a not uncommon presentation in the field of ID)?

Reminiscence therapy

Reminiscence therapy involves the discussion of past activities, experiences or events with the aid of familiar items, photographs or music. Often it involves memories of earlier life events being recalled and discussed, rather than people being asked to recall events from the same day. Due to methodological issues with regard to research, there is limited information available on whether reminiscence therapy is actually beneficial either cognitively or behaviourally (Spector *et al.* 2000b). Further studies are required to assess the role of reminiscence therapy in the treatment of DAD in adults with ID.

Cognitive behavioural therapy

With the growing awareness of non-cognitive psychological and behavioural symptoms of DAD, psychological techniques for treating associated anxiety or depressive symptoms have been developed. There is some evidence that cognitive behavioural intervention can reduce the burden on carers in the general population (Akkerman and Ostwald 2004). Progressive relaxation techniques are used to reduce anxiety and agitation. Depressive mood may be alleviated by discussing pleasant events on a regular basis. As with other non-pharmacological techniques, further research and clinical evidence is required prior to the implementation of cognitive behavioural therapy in older adults with ID and dementia.

Treatment of physical problems

Declining physical health is an integral part of DAD (*see* Chapter 4). Common areas of decline include mobility, swallowing, sphincter control and maintenance of body weight. The involvement of the occupational therapist and the speech and language therapist in undertaking the appropriate assessment of motor and process skills and of swallowing and in providing practical help for carers is an important part of the multi-disciplinary care programme.

As mentioned previously, while the underlying DAD is treated with anti-dementia medication and/or psychological interventions, other groups of drugs are used to target specific symptoms. The different drug groups and the specific psychopathologies that they are used to treat are reviewed below.

Antipsychotic medication

Although recently the focus of drug therapy has been to treat the underlying AD process, historically drug treatment has been primarily aimed at reducing the non-cognitive psychopathological aspects of DAD. A wide spectrum of behavioural and psychological symptoms of dementia occurs in adults with DAD. These symptoms include aggression, anxiety, agitation, perceptual changes (hallucinations and delusions), mood changes (depression and irritability) and disturbance of biological functions (e.g. the sleep cycle) (*see* Chapter 4). Often more than one problem will occur at the same time in adults with DAD. These symptoms can cause considerable concern to both the patient and their carers.

Antipsychotic medication to treat mental disorders – including dementia – has now been available for at least 50 years. Conventional antipsychotics work by blocking dopamine receptors in the brain, and are used principally to treat problematic behaviours, delusions and hallucinations, and irritability (Lawlor 2004). A wide range of antipsychotic drugs are available (*see* Table 7.6). The majority of the atypical antipsychotic drugs work by interfering with dopaminergic transmission in the brain by blocking dopamine D_2 receptors. Some can also affect cholinergic, α-adrenergic, histaminergic and serotonergic receptors.

It is important to determine the specific problem that is being addressed and to understand the relative benefits of the different types of medication which can be prescribed. Withdrawal of drugs after long-term therapy should always be gradual and monitored in order to avoid the risk of acute withdrawal syndromes or recurrence of symptoms.

To date, antipsychotic drugs remain the first-line pharmacological treatment for behavioural disorders associated with DAD, even in the absence of evidence from randomised controlled drug trials supporting the role of conventional antipsychotics in the treatment of behavioural and psychological symptoms in DAD. The benefit may not be dose related, and there may be no significant differences between the different conventional antipsychotics (Schneider *et al.* 1990). The newer atypical neuroleptics are reported to be more selective in their neurotransmitter action, and subsequently have fewer extrapyramidal and sedative side-effects. Recent randomised controlled trials in the general population have suggested that the atypical antipsychotics can significantly reduce behavioural and psychological symptoms in adults with DAD. Tariot *et al.* (2004) conducted a

Table 7.6 Common neuroleptic drugs

Conventional	Atypical
Haloperidol	Amisulpiride
Chorpromazine	Risperidone
Trifluoperazine	Olanzapine
Flupenthixol	Quetiapine
Promazine	Aripiprazole
Pimozide	Clozapine
Thioridazine	Zotepine

12-week study of risperidone in patients with DAD and found a dose-related improvement in psychosis and agitation. Olanzapine and quetiapine have been demonstrated to reduce agitation, aggression and psychosis in individuals with DAD (Scharre and Chang 2002; Schatz 2003). The effects of antipsychotic treatment on quality of life require further investigation.

Side-effects, particularly in elderly people who may also be physically quite frail, remain a cause for concern. The initiation of antipsychotic medication should be undertaken slowly with gradual increases in dosage, and where possible the long-term usage of such drugs should be avoided. By far the most troublesome side-effects are extrapyramidal symptoms. They occur frequently with the piperazine phenothiazines (chlorpromazine, trifluoperazine), the butyrophenones (benperidol and haloperidol) and the depot preparations. Extrapyramidal symptoms include the following:

- parkinsonian symptoms (tremor, slowness)
- dystonia (abnormal face and body movements) and dyskinesia
- akathisia (restlessness)
- tardive dyskinesia (rhythmic, involuntary movements of the tongue, face and jaw).

Parkinsonian symptoms remit if the drug is withdrawn and may be suppressed by the administration of antimuscarinic drugs (e.g. procyclidine). In addition to the extrapyramidal side-effects, postural hypotension, falls, sedation, arrhythmias, blurred vision and acute confusional state are of particular concern in adults with DAD. Recently, the atypical antipsychotic drugs (risperidone and olanzapine) have been associated with a two- to threefold increased risk of a stroke and a two- to threefold increase in mortality in elderly people with dementia in the general population (Wooltorton 2002, 2004). However, not all researchers have found an increased risk (Gill *et al.* 2005). Any risk is thought to be greatest in the very elderly (over 80 years of age) and in individuals with diabetes, obesity, hypertension, smoking or heart disease. In the UK, the Committee on Safety of Medicines advised that these drugs should not be used to treat behavioural symptoms in dementia (Insau and Lawley 2004). However, the opinion of the Royal College of Psychiatrists (2004) is that these drugs are still worth using in some circumstances, particularly when alternative drug treatments may have similar or worse side-effects and non-pharmacological approaches are unsuitable. As there is no information available at present about the risks in older adults with ID, it is pertinent to bear in mind that the risk of a stroke cannot be excluded in adults with ID who have DAD and are started on atypical antipsychotic medication. Drug treatment should be targeted at a specific symptom, initiated at a low dose, titrated gradually, and continued for a limited time period.

Antidepressants

Depressive symptoms may not only be part of the psychopathology of DAD but can also occur prior to the presentation of cognitive decline (Lyketsos and Lee 2004). The symptoms and signs of depression that are seen in adults with DAD are not too dissimilar to those seen in younger people with depression, namely low mood, tearfulness, disturbed sleep, poor appetite, apathy and agitation. There can be more marked episodes of aggression, confusion and restlessness. The different classes of antidepressant are listed in Table 7.7. Antidepressants usually work by blocking the reuptake of neurotransmitters in the synaptic cleft, thereby increasing their availability to the postsynaptic receptors, and increasing neuronal function. Findings for the general population vary, but around 5–15% of adults with DAD can suffer from a major depressive episode. Up to 50% of individuals with dementia may present with depressive features at any one time. Tsiouris and Patti (1997) and Geldmacher *et al.* (1997) highlighted the overlap between a depressive episode and dementia in adults with ID. The importance of prompt treatment with antidepressants was highlighted by both studies.

Gedye (1991) tested the effectiveness of a low-dose antidepressant (trazodone) together with a serotonin-enhancing diet in reducing aggression in an adult with DS who showed signs of DAD. The benefit was robustly demonstrated using an 'on–off–on again' design with detailed recording for nearly 4 months. The level of aggression decreased by 96%.

Although the general principle is that non-pharmacological treatment should be used initially, antidepressants can be beneficial. It must be borne in mind that antidepressants can take 2–3 weeks to show benefit, and full recovery may not be evident until 2–3 months on a therapeutic dose of medication (Tune 1998).

Anti-anxiety medication

Increased anxiety, tension, agitation and distress are known to occur in people with dementia, and a number of drugs have been used to reduce this anxiety. These are principally benzodiazepines and chlor derivatives (choral hydrate), which potenti-

Table 7.7 Different classes of antidepressant medication

Selective serotonin reuptake inhibitors	Serotonin noradrenaline reuptake inhibitors	Tricyclic and related antidepressants	Monoamine oxidase inhibitors
Fluoxetine	Venlafaxine	Amitriptyline	Phenelzine
Paroxetine		Dothiepin	Tranylcypromine
Citalopram		Lofepramine	
Sertraline		Imipramine	
		Trazodone	

ate the inhibitory action of γ-aminobutyric acid. Other drugs that have been used include buspirone and beta-blockers (e.g. propranolol). The latter drugs are less sedative and addictive than benzodiazepines, and tolerance does not develop. Benzodiazepines have side-effects such as sedation and unsteadiness, and can impair cognitive function if given at too high a dose. Subsequent to initial treatment with these drugs their use needs to be monitored frequently. Where possible, anxiolytic drugs should not be prescribed for more than 4–6 weeks.

Anti-epileptics

Late-onset seizures are common in adults with ID and DAD (*see* Chapter 4). Once a person with DAD has developed seizures, the aim of any treatment is to prevent further seizures by maintaining an effective dose of anti-epileptic drugs. A gradual increase in dose is necessary until seizures are controlled or side-effects occur. Most anti-epileptics can be given twice daily. Therapy with more than one anti-epileptic drug may be necessary, but should only occur when monotherapy with several alternative drugs has proved ineffective. Combination therapy enhances toxicity, and drug interactions may occur between the different anti-epileptic drugs. Abrupt withdrawal of anti-epileptics (particularly the barbiturates and benzodiazepines) can cause severe rebound seizures. The dose should be reduced in gradual increments, and this process can take up to a year. In patients who are receiving several anti-epileptic drugs, only one drug should be withdrawn at a time. For adults with DAD it is likely that once anti-epileptic drug therapy has been started it will continue until death. The most commonly used anti-epileptic drugs are listed in Box 7.1.

Box 7.1 Commonly used anti-epileptic drugs

Carbamazepine
Ethosuximide
Gabapentin
Lamotrigine
Levetiracetam
Oxcarbazepine
Phenobarbital
Primidone
Phenytoin
Topiramate
Sodium valproate
Vigabatrin

The initiation of anti-epileptic medication should follow similar guidelines to those for younger adults with ID who have epilepsy. Greater caution is needed when initiating medication, as some of the side-effects of these drugs may include sedation or ataxia. Anticonvulsant medication has been reported to reduce behavioural problems (Barry *et al.* 2004) and may therefore have secondary benefits in adults with DAD.

Management of insomnia

A detailed assessment of the pattern, duration and severity of disturbed sleep should be documented. Underlying causes should be sought through a careful medical examination before it is assumed that the cause is dementia. For example, has there been a change in the bedtime routine or is there excessive noise? A number of non-pharmacological treatments are available which may benefit sleep patterns (*see* Box 7.2).

Box 7.2 Non-pharmacological interventions for insomnia

Avoid excessive use of stimulants, such as coffee and tea, in the evening.
Maintain a regular sleep routine.
Minimise excessive noise.
Avoid disturbing the patient in order to dispense their medication.
Encourage the patient to go to the toilet prior to going to bed.
Avoid daytime sleeping.
Ensure that the room is neither too cold nor too warm.

Psychological treatments (e.g. relaxation therapy, behavioural intervention) have been demonstrated to regulate the sleep–wake cycle in older adults in the general population. Such techniques have a limited role to play in older adults with ID with dementia. Occasionally pharmacological medication may be required. Hypnotic medication should only be used if other measures have been unsuccessful and the sleep disturbance is having a significant impact on the life of the individual and/or their carers. The dose should be low initially, given on alternate days and gradually increased. The commonest types of hypnotics used are listed in Box 7.3.

Box 7.3 Commonly used hypnotics

Benzodiazepines
Diazepam
Temazepam
Lorazepam
Nitrazepam
Flurazepam
Lormetazepam

Z drugs
Zaleplon
Zolpidem
Zopiclone

Chloral derivatives
Chloral hydrate
Triclofos sodium
Clormethiazole

The two most commonly used drug groups (benzodiazepines and Z drugs) work by enhancing neuronal inhibition by γ-aminobutyric acid (GABA) by binding to specific GABA receptors in the brain. Hypnotics have a rapid onset of action (30–90 minutes), and the Z drugs have a shorter duration of action than the benzodiazepines. Hypnotics can aid all types of sleep disturbance, but tolerance can develop after a few weeks. The drugs should be stopped gradually, as abrupt cessation can lead to rebound insomnia. Long-term use should be avoided.

There are a number of adverse effects associated with hypnotic drug use. Older people with dementia are particularly susceptible to side-effects due to impaired drug metabolism and possible drug interactions. Over-sedation and daytime hangover effects can present as further impaired cognitive function, unsteadiness, falls, confusion and apathy.

Management of behavioural problems

The assessment and management of behavioural problems in older adults with ID who have dementia is best undertaken using a multi-disciplinary approach, including psychiatrists, general physicians, psychologists, community nurses, social workers and carers. Often the optimum management of the agitation and/or aggression will involve a multi-therapeutic approach rather than a single form of therapy. In addition, any intervention may take time, and indeed the patient's condition may deteriorate further before there is improvement. Both ongoing support for carers and monitoring by professionals are required.

For any given behavioural problem, a number of general principles apply.

1 Identify the specific problem and behaviour that need to be treated.
2 Evaluate the environment with regard to changes that could be made in order to reduce the behaviour.
3 If necessary, initiate appropriate psychopharmacological medication.
4 Review the situation on a regular ongoing basis.

It is important to highlight a specific problem, such as hitting, biting or screaming, rather than to try to treat 'agitation' or 'aggression'. A change to the environment and how carers respond to difficult behaviours should initially be tried. Improving communication and avoiding over-stimulation may reduce problematic behaviour. Psychopharmacological medication can be used, but this may involve initially treating any secondary psychiatric disorder (e.g. depression). Consideration should be given to preventing interaction with other medication and to monitoring the patient for side-effects. Antipsychotic medication has often been used to treat behavioural disturbance, with no marked advantage being apparent for any particular type of drug. The most commonly used conventional drugs include chlorpromazine, thioridazine and haloperidol. Antidepressants, beta-blockers and anxiolytics (particularly benzodiazepines and buspirone) have all been used and have some beneficial effect. However, these drugs can accumulate in the bloodstream over time, increasing the risk of falls and sedation, as well as confusion in elderly people. Occasionally augmentation therapies are used, whereby antipsychotic medication is given alongside an anxiolytic or antidepressant. Caution is required in such cases.

Management of agitation and aggression

Agitation and aggression can have many causes in elderly people with ID and dementia (*see* Box 7.4), and several of these factors may overlap with each other. In some cases no particular cause will be found.

Box 7.4 Common causes of behavioural problems

Progressive dementia *per se*
An associated medical disorder
Side-effects of medication
Specific or generalised discomfort
An associated psychiatric illness
Sleep disturbance
Environmental factors
Communication difficulties
Carer stress
Physical abuse

Dementia in Alzheimer's disease is due to changes within the brain leading to atrophy and loss of neurotransmitter chemicals. Specific areas of the brain that control or influence mood and/or behaviour may be affected, as well as the areas that control memory and speech. For example, agitation, changes in personality and aggression are particularly associated with the frontal cortex and antero-temporal region. The generalised atrophy that is seen in DAD will be associated with disruption of the normal functioning of the neurotransmitter circulation, and this could lead to agitation and behavioural problems. Older dementing adults, as they become more weak and frail, are particularly susceptible to the effects of a concurrent medical illness (e.g. chest infection, urinary tract infection, dehydration). Physical ill health superimposed on the underlying dementia can lead to increased confusion. A concurrent medical illness may present as agitation or behavioural problems. Sensory impairment, particularly poor hearing and loss of vision (both of which are common in older adults with DS), may lead to a person with dementia further misunderstanding and misreading their environment, resulting in increased agitation, restlessness and aggression.

The assessment of agitation and behavioural problems follows a three-step process.

1 Obtain a description of the problem.
2 Determine its severity.
3 Identify possible underlying factors.

An assessment using an 'ABC chart' can often provide a detailed picture of the problem. A particular antecedent that triggers the agitation and/or aggression may be identified. An assessment with regard to an antecedent would involve obtaining information about the particular time of the day when the behaviour occurs, the particular environment in which it occurs, and possibly whether it occurs in the company of a particular person. Have there been any recent changes in the person's environment that could have led to problems? Are the behaviours associated with any underlying mental illness, such as paranoia, depression or delirium? The assessment of the behaviour would include specific information about the exact nature of the problem that is causing concern. How frequent and severe is the problem? Has it led to any injuries to the person him- or herself or to others? Is the behaviour getting worse? Are a number of behaviours present and do they interact with and exacerbate each other? What is the impact of the behaviour on other clients and on staff members? What are the consequences of the behaviour? How is the behaviour managed? What helps to reduce the behaviour? Are there any reinforcers of the behaviour? And what is the impact of the behaviour on the person's quality of life?

A detailed multi-disciplinary assessment may be necessary. Laboratory tests may be required in order to exclude a physical disorder (e.g. urinary analysis to rule out urinary tract infection). A detailed health screen to rule out any possible causes of pain (e.g. toothache, constipation), or deterioration in hearing or vision should be undertaken. Prescribed medication should be reviewed. A number of behavioural rating scales are available and these could be used to monitor the behaviour and agitation over time.

Elderly people in general are susceptible to the side-effects or interactions of prescribed medication, especially psychotropic drugs such as anti-dementia drugs or neuroleptic sedating drugs. If these drugs are initiated too quickly, prescribed at too high a dose or prescribed concurrently, exacerbation of confusion can result, leading to behavioural problems. Changes in a person's environment, particularly frequent changes in care staff or in daytime activities, can cause unnecessary anxiety leading to agitation and/or aggression. Carers themselves may not understand or be fully aware of the clinical features of dementia, and may misread or misunderstand behaviours associated with this progressive neurode-generative disease. This may lead to inappropriate handling/management of the person with dementia, with resulting aggression. For example, disruption of the sleep cycle (a common feature of dementia) may lead to a person being awake at night. Carers may misinterpret this as the person being 'naughty', and insist that they return to and remain in bed. The person with dementia may not understand why they are being asked to do this, which may result in their displaying physical aggression towards the carer.

Environmental and carer interventions

Changes to the environment to enable carers to cope with the substantial needs of a person with dementia have been briefly mentioned above. The particular needs of carers will be discussed in detail in Chapter 8.

Summary

On the basis of evidence for the general population and for the ID population, it is reasonable to treat older adults with DAD in the ID population with anti-dementia medication. However, the risks of prescribing medication do need to be balanced against possible side-effects, such as falls, sedation and gastrointestinal upsets, which may be of particular concern in the elderly, who will probably already be taking a number of other drugs. It is important that treatment is initiated at a low dosage, with gradual increases over time and close monitoring. In the UK, the National Institute for Clinical Excellence (2001) has set a number of guidelines for the use of anti-dementia drugs. These include the following:

1 The diagnosis of DAD should be made by a specialist.
2 Baseline assessment and monitoring using a number of tools should be part of the management plan.
3 A specialist should initiate treatment and assess the response to treatment.

These guidelines should be adhered to when treating adults with ID with DAD.

Concurrent with anti-dementia drug therapy there should be ongoing management of comorbid conditions, treatment of behavioural and mood disorders using pharmacological and non-pharmacological approaches, and provision of support and resources for both the patient and their caregivers (*see* Chapter 8). Multi-disciplinary teamworking with close monitoring enables optimum care to be provided. However, the impact on quality of life of interventional therapy for DAD has yet to be determined.

Chapter 8

Carer needs and support services

Carer burden

It is now well recognised that family carers experience a considerable degree of stress while looking after a person with dementia in Alzheimer's disease (DAD) (Wenger *et al.* 2002). Confusion, behavioural change, psychiatric symptoms and physical ill health can all take their toll on carers (both family members and paid carers). Although many professional agencies can provide support, this is usually limited to weekdays from 9.00a.m. to 5.00p.m. However, considerable stress can be experienced by carers in the evenings, at night-time and at weekends, when access to services is limited. Family carers are often elderly parents who themselves have considerable psychological and physical health needs. The type, severity and duration of stress experienced by carers are determined by a combination of the physical and emotional demands on the carer. This in turn is dependent on the severity of the dementia, the coping skills available to the carers, and the level of ongoing support from professionals, other family member, friends and neighbours.

Family carers in the general population are reported to be at increased risk of depression and anxiety while caring for a person with dementia (Goodman 1986). Family members can become exhausted, and as well as feeling anxious and depressed they may have strong feelings of guilt and grief. With regard to the ID population, adults with dementia are often resident in community group homes and looked after by paid carers, who can work shift patterns and share their responsibilities with older carers, thereby reducing the carer burden. It is important that as part of the management of individuals with dementia, ongoing support is provided for carers, particularly at an early stage. Access to respite and day-care services can significantly reduce carer stress by allowing carers to have private time to undertake personal duties and activities and giving them a break from the demands of caregiving. The importance of care burden should not be overlooked, as in extreme cases physical and emotional abuse of patients with dementia has been reported.

Caregivers often assume an overwhelming responsibility and burden day after day, sometimes for several years, while caring for a person with dementia in their family home. Time is spent on ensuring good hygiene, providing ingestible meals, monitoring the patient's medication, attending appointments, engaging the patient in activities, and being constantly aware of issues of safety. Care provision is therefore a full-time occupation, often 24 hours a day, 7 days a week.

Oliver *et al.* (2000) demonstrated that adults with DS who showed cognitive deterioration had more adverse life experiences than those with no cognitive deterioration. Specific areas included leisure, relationships and opportunities. Furthermore, caregivers' difficulties were greater if they were caring for individuals with cognitive decline. The authors suggested that the changing role of caregivers could influence the cognitive decline seen in adults with DS. McCarron *et al.* (2002) investigated the time spent by caregivers with adults with DS who had DAD, using the Caregiver Activity Survey–Intellectual Disability Questionnaire (CAS-IDQ), which measures time spent by professional caregivers assisting people with DS and dementia. A total of 30 individuals with DS were selected, of whom 14 subjects did not have dementia. These were matched with 16 subjects who had dementia according to *ICD-10* criteria (World Health Organization 1992). The study found that over a 24-hour period, the overall time spent by carers of adults with dementia was greater than that for carers of those without dementia (9 hours versus 2.35 hours). There was no difference in the time spent by carers of adults with mid-stage and end-stage dementia, although the nature and tasks of caregiving did change as the dementia progressed. The authors confirmed the need for services to be able to adapt to changes in their ageing population.

Whitehouse *et al.* (2000) assessed carer staff knowledge and attitudes towards people with ID who had dementia. In total, 21 members of the care staff working in a home for people with ID over the age of 65 years were assessed. A number of questionnaires were used to assess caregivers' knowledge and understanding of dementia. Reported signs of dementia included forgetfulness, confusion, withdrawal, irritation/agitation, aggression, behavioural changes, disorientation, constant frustration, accusations and memory problems. However, only forgetfulness was reported by more than half of the carers, and the vast majority of the signs were reported by fewer than five caregivers. The study highlighted the fact that staff working with adults with ID who have dementia require further education and training, and that services need to address these issues.

It must also be borne in mind that in the field of ID the vast majority of family and paid carers do not routinely care for older adults with dementia. If a person does develop DAD with resulting cognitive decline, physical decline and behavioural problems, particularly aggression, wandering and agitation, this can cause considerable resentment among carers. In turn this can lead to carers withdrawing from active involvement. Carers may find it easier to undertake their day-to-day activities but avoid any communication with the person with dementia. This can inadvertently generate an environment in which there is rapid deterioration and poor support. As part of the dementia 'work-up', professionals should assess the type and degree of communication that is taking place.

It may be important that a member of the multi-disciplinary team is given responsibility to assess carer stress and to monitor any carer burden as part of the care package. Specific signs of stress may include feeling generally tired, angry or anxious, not sleeping, and a decline in physical health. It is not uncommon for an older carer to say 'but only I know how to look after my daughter/son'. It is also not uncommon for elderly family carers to deny any feelings of being burdened, and to deny the need for personal support. Such emotions may reflect underlying feelings of deep anger and guilt. However, it is often these carers who require the most support. And carers do require support, given with considerable empathy. They must be allowed to have time to speak to someone and verbalise their feelings.

In some regions of the UK such a role is taken on by a Dementia Nurse Specialist, who can respond quickly to concerns expressed by carers, provide ongoing good-quality care and support, foster positive attitudes towards caring for a person with dementia, and develop new skills in terms of training and development.

Caregiving interventions

A number of studies in the general population have demonstrated the benefits of intervention measures for carers of adults with dementia (Brodaty *et al.* 1994, McCarron 1999; Marriott *et al.* 2000). The types of interventions that have been used include providing basic information on DAD for carers, development of support groups, carer training on how to manage behavioural problems, ongoing counselling, and advice on how to better access regular respite services.

Physical changes to the environment can aid the carer for a person with dementia. These include environmental changes to improve sensory stimulation and safety (e.g. better lighting), improving the layout of the building to improve orientation and mobility, and making adaptations to the bathroom, toilet, dining room and kitchen to allow the person to maintain his or her domestic skills (*see* Table 8.1) (Day *et al.* 2000). Such interventions can also reduce the care burden and improve the quality of life of the person with DAD (Dooley and Hinojosa 2004). Furthermore, it is known that in the general population increased carer intervention can delay admission to a nursing home (Mittelman *et al.* 1996). Research investigating future developments in services for the elderly with ID and dementia is urgently needed (McCarthy and Mullan 1996).

It is important for carers to continue activities that maintain the self-esteem of individuals with ID who have dementia (McCarron 1999). For example, it is important that mealtimes remain a social occasion, and that adequate time is allowed for the person to finish their meal. Routines should be simplified,

Table 8.1 Carer interventions

Type	Comments
Education	Giving information to carers about the diagnosis, the disease, the outcome, the available resources and treatment is important. General advice on maintaining day-to-day skills (e.g. clothes being laid out in order to encourage dressing)
Support	Carers require ongoing support with regard to how to manage a person with a progressive disease and how to communicate better with the person with dementia (e.g. learn to speak calmly and with a louder voice). Questions and requests should be made in simple language, and one at a time with enough time given for the person to respond
Environment	Changes in the environment in terms of safety adaptations can reduce carer stress. Advice on household hazards (e.g. doors being locked appropriately, bathing time). The engagement of carers and patients in outdoor activities can maintain morale. Future plans should involve long-term placement, and respite care should be considered
Access to services	Carers may want to access social service agencies for increased day care, respite care, home help, or occupational and physiotherapy support

attention should be given to the likes and dislikes of the person, and assistance and advice should be made available if necessary. Carers can also maintain communication by establishing eye contact, reducing background noise, and communicating with visual aids (e.g. photographs) (Woods 1998).

It is often difficult for family carers to decide at what point their loved one with dementia may require alternative long-term care. Severe dementia, frequent accidents, ongoing behavioural problems and high levels of carer stress are common factors that lead to a transfer to a long-term care facility. Very occasionally, concern about neglect or abuse may trigger services intervention. The issue of transfer to a long-term care facility is difficult and needs to be raised with considerable empathy, particularly with family carers. The benefits of long-term care for both the patient and the carer should be highlighted. Where possible the transfer to long-term care should be planned in advance and be part of the ongoing care plan. The patient should be allowed to take personal items with them to the new residence, and bedrooms should be made as homely as possible. Carers should be allowed to visit and continue to participate in the care (e.g. by helping with feeding).

Services

With an increasing number of adults with ID surviving into old age, it is becoming apparent that there is inadequate provision of appropriate services (Davidson *et al.* 2004). There is still a scarcity of information about the growth of the ageing ID population, the health and social needs of these individuals, and the most appropriate services for them. Ideally a national survey of the number of ageing individuals and their specific health and social needs, together with discussions on future services, is needed. Health promotion and the prevention of age-related diseases are areas that are noticeably overlooked in the ageing ID population. However, during the last two decades there have been considerable developments in community services for people with ID as a whole, which should allow older adults with ID to access the health promotion services that are available to the general population. Community health services, psychiatric services, social and residential care providers, the private sector and voluntary organisations have all contributed to a significant move away from institutionalised care towards a more community-based form of care. At times it has appeared that service development for older adults with ID has been lost in the general transfer of services into the community. It is only recently that attention has been given to providing a more specific service for older adults with ID.

The optimum management of DAD in adults with ID depends on multi-disciplinary and multi-agency services working closely together. In the UK, services are structured as *primary health services* where patients can access the National Health Service, usually through their general practitioner, and *secondary specialist services*, where more intensive health services can be accessed (e.g. memory clinics, hospital inpatient care). The level of access for older adults with ID to a specialist dementia service remains variable across the UK, but is generally poor. It remains imperative that individuals who may have dementia are referred to the specialist dementia service at an early stage, where they can be evaluated for possible dementia and an appropriate management plan can be formulated and implemented.

Greater support and care can be provided by the specialist service than by the primary service. A diagnosis of DAD should certainly be made by the specialist service and not by a general physician. Furthermore, with the advent of anti-dementia therapy, the earlier the treatment is initiated the more likely it is that there will be a benefit. For the ID population it is best practice for the primary health service to refer all older people with evidence of intellectual and/or adaptive decline to the ageing ID service. Whenever possible this referral should be made to a physician with a specialist interest in ageing issues in the ID population.

In practice in the UK, adults with ID who have dementia are often referred to a number of specialists, who may include geriatricians, old age psychiatrists, neurologists and ID psychiatrists. A number of regions across the UK may have memory clinics either for older adults in the general population or specifically for older adults with ID. In the UK the National Service Framework (NSF) for Older Adults has been developed to improve standard care and set national guidelines for health and social care across the UK. The NSF for older people has been developed to ensure prompt diagnosis, easy and quick access to specialist services, early initiation of the appropriate treatment and the provision of ongoing carer advice and support. The effect of the implementation of the NSF has not yet been evaluated.

Multi-disciplinary team

As was mentioned earlier, effective inter-disciplinary working and greater communication between the primary and secondary services are necessary if a high-quality service is to be provided. Table 8.2 lists the main members of the ID multi-disciplinary team.

Table 8.2 Members of the multi-disciplinary team

Professional	Principal work
Psychiatrist	Medical doctor with professional training in field of ID. Able to diagnosis and treat dementia principally with medication. Able to access other professionals
Community nurse	Mental health trained nurse. Coordinates care for patients in specialist service. Monitors ongoing treatment in the community. Helps to liaise between different services and provides advice and support for carers
Psychologist	Able to undertake psychiatric assessments to measure cognitive and social functioning. Coordinates and supervises various psychological and behavioural treatments
Occupational therapist	Provides physical and psychiatric treatment to maintain mild level of functioning in the community. Able to access adaptations to the family home and assess levels of safety
Social worker	Provides community care support. Able to provide information about other residential services and advise on benefits
General practitioner	Medical doctor who is first port of call for patient in the community. Able to monitor and prescribe medication and continue to assess for any ongoing physical conditions. Through the primary care service is able to provide other services (e.g. incontinence nurse)

Components of an ID dementia service

Community services

For a community-based dementia service to function effectively and appropriately, it requires a multi-disciplinary ID team. This includes a psychiatrist, community ID nurse, social workers, psychologist, occupational health therapist, speech and language therapist, physiotherapist and administrative staff. Such a team can provide adequate assessment, ensure effective delivery of any treatment, reduce carer stress, and improve the quality of life of the person with ID and dementia.

It remains uncertain how a community team can operate most effectively. Should referrals be on an 'open referrals system' (i.e. any individual can refer a person to the team), or should they only be made by a medical practitioner? Should the initial assessment always be made by a doctor (e.g. a psychiatrist), or should other professionals undertake the initial assessments (e.g. nurses). Evidence from the general population would suggest that an open referral system and referrals seen by any member of the team represent the most efficient way of managing new referrals.

Respite

As was discussed earlier, caring for an elderly person with ID who has dementia causes considerable stress to family carers and significantly impairs their social activities. Providing respite is one means whereby carers can be enabled to take a break from their caring responsibilities and still continue an active social life. Admission to a respite care unit can also allow further assessments of the severity of dementia to take place, as well as monitoring for side-effects of newly prescribed medication. The increased disruption to the person with dementia needs to be balanced against the benefits to the carers.

Day care

Day-care facilities for older adults with dementia are usually part of the generic services for people with ID. It is more beneficial for older adults with dementia to have specific and separate day care. Such facilities can allow detailed assessment and monitoring of patients to take place with regard to a whole range of daily activities in a way that may not be possible in generic day-care facilities. Furthermore, elderly individuals with dementia require a quieter and less 'busy' environment.

Memory clinics

In the UK there are a limited number of memory clinics for people with ID. However, in the general population these are now widely available, and approximately 30 clinics are well established nationwide. The vast majority work on a multi-disciplinary basis. Although many were initially set up as research centres, they have now become part of the mainstream service provision. Memory clinics usually have seven aims:

1 diagnosis
2 treatment
3 monitoring of dementia over time

4 the provision of non-pharmacological interventions
5 planning for the future
6 educating carers and professionals
7 participation in research.

With a focus on the specific use of anti-dementia drug therapies, and an emphasis on the importance of a detailed 'work-up', several dementia clinics for ID are being established across the UK, and they can aid the development of a wider dementia service. A general memory clinic care pathway is shown in Figure 8.1.

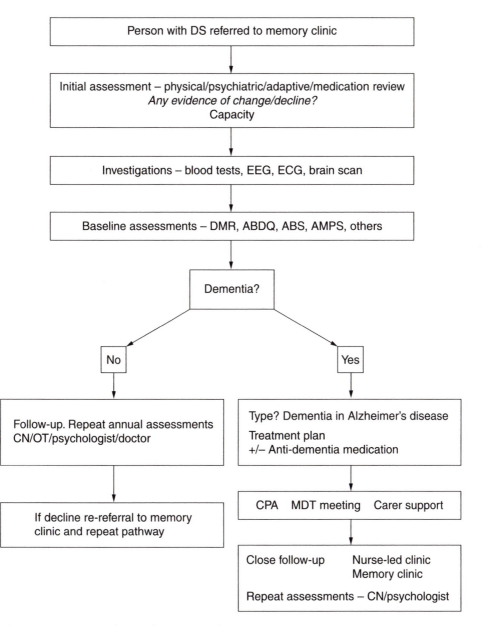

Figure 8.1 Down syndrome dementia pathway.

Monitoring services: nurse-led clinics

There is a considerable lack of research on the monitoring of older adults with ID and dementia on a long-term basis. Further studies are needed to determine the service utilisation, the benefits of anti-dementia medication, support for carers, and improvement of quality of life for dementia sufferers. Nurse-led clinics offer one way of maintaining ongoing regular and frequent contact with individuals with dementia. After the initial detailed assessment and management plan has been formulated in the memory clinic, a dementia nurse specialist can undertake much of the ongoing care. Such clinics are still in their infancy, but are likely to be a valuable addition to the provision of high-quality care.

Long-term care

There is still considerable uncertainty about the most appropriate type of long-term care for a person with ID who develops DAD. By default various care systems are in place, including families with whom these individuals are living, residential care providers and generic nursing-home facilities. All of these lack the necessary funding and training to provide 24-hour care where the needs will vary from those associated with mild dementia to the more complex needs of late-stage dementia. Specialist long-stay units for elderly people with ID, commissioned by ID services, are being developed. These units have specially trained staff with experience in caring for elderly people with ID, modified environments to allow more effective management of challenging behaviour and the associated physical needs of DAD, medical care provided by a specialist dementia team, and a prevailing ethos of the need for high-quality care for very vulnerable individuals. A balance needs to be achieved between the need to maintain an individual's autonomy and quality of life and the need to ensure safety and minimise risk of injury.

Irrespective of which care system is in place, it is important that care is planned and that it is agreed by all of the parties involved. Far too often a crisis occurs that leads to unplanned and poorly made decisions which can exaggerate the underlying dementing process. Further research is needed to evaluate the different types of long-term care. However, international guidelines have been published that provide guidance on stage-related care management of DAD and suggestions for service development (Janicki et al. 1996).

Summary

The carer burden is often not managed appropriately in the field of ID, and is often overlooked in the pursuit of a clinical diagnosis of DAD. Frequently family carers are elderly and have their own healthcare needs. Providing 24-hour support for a person with a progressive neurodegenerative disorder is extremely burdensome, and it is the responsibility of healthcare providers to make available the appropriate support to reduce such stress. Different forms of intervention can be provided by the multi-disciplinary team, not only to improve the quality of life of the person with dementia, but also – importantly – to improve the quality of life of the carer.

High-quality services for adults with ID and dementia remain primarily in their infancy. The development of memory clinics, older adult day-care services and more integrated services suggests that progress, albeit slow, is being made. Further research is needed to formally determine the most clinically effective and cost-effective service for older adults with ID who develop DAD.

Chapter 9

Future prospects

Older adults with ID form a minority group of the general population, but because of their complex and special needs they require an intensive and integrated specialist service. Over the next two decades the population of elderly adults with ID will grow rapidly. These individuals are susceptible to a range of psychiatric disorders, in particular dementia in Alzheimer's disease (DAD). With the recent closure of long-stay hospitals and resettlement of older adults into the community, the primary health service requires ongoing support from the specialist services to provide optimum care.

There is still limited information on how people with ID actually 'age'. Do people with Down syndrome (DS) suffer from premature ageing? Is the ageing process the same irrespective of the underlying cause of the ID, or is ageing only affected by, for example, chromosomal syndromes? Certainly an association between DS and AD has now been established, but limited research data are available about the possible association between ID generally and dementia. The effects of age-associated functional decline (normal ageing) and its relationship to dementia remain an area for further investigation.

The development of pharmacological agents to treat DAD in adults with ID has been one of the most significant developments of recent times. Undoubtedly over the next decade further research will be made available regarding the efficacy of these drugs, clinical differences between the available drug types, and their roles in disease prevention and in modifying the underlying disease process. Temporary clinical relief has been demonstrated in adults with DS who develop DAD, but long-term studies are needed to determine the effects on quality of life and the cost-effectiveness of treatment.

The accurate diagnosis of DAD in adults with ID is still an area of concern, but future developments in the identification of biological markers may help to resolve this issue. Macrocytosis, free radical changes, plasma amyloid load and neuroimaging abnormalities are areas of ongoing and future interest. Biological aspects of DAD in adults with DS will be the focus of future research.

With the molecular mapping of chromosome 21, the genetic association between DS and AD will advance considerably from the present position, namely that adults with DS have triplication of the amyloid precursor protein (APP) gene. Identification of polymorphisms of the APP gene, and isolation of promoter and other regulatory genes in the critical region of DS will enhance our understanding of the aetiology of AD in the DS population. Associated stem-cell research remains an exciting area of future development.

Service and clinical developments are ongoing. In 2001, a number of international researchers and clinicians met and developed a working group on dementia care practices (Wilkinson and Janicki 2002). They produced the *Edinburgh principles*, which can be summarised as follows.

1   Adopt an operational philosophy that promotes the utmost quality of life of people with ID affected by dementia, and whenever possible base services and support practices on a person-centred approach.
2   Affirm that individual strengths, capabilities, skills and wishes should be the overriding consideration in any decision making for or by people with ID affected by dementia.
3   Involve the individual, his or her family, and other close supports in all phases of assessment and services planning and provision for the person with an ID-affected dementia.
4   Ensure that appropriate diagnostic, assessment and intervention services and resources are available to meet the individual needs and support the healthy ageing of people with ID affected by dementia.
5   Plan and provide support and services that optimise remaining in the chosen home and community of adults with ID affected by dementia.
6   Ensure that people with ID affected by dementia have the same access to appropriate services and support as is afforded to other people in the general population affected by dementia.
7   Ensure that generic, co-operative and proactive strategic planning across relevant policy, provider and advocacy groups involves consideration of the current and future needs of adults with ID affected by dementia.

The universal implementation of these principles would go a long way towards ensuring that older adults with ID receive the care they deserve and age healthily. This includes the right to a healthy lifestyle, a healthy living environment, a positive mental attitude towards ageing, a positive support network, and safety, security and stability.

Now that we have entered the twenty-first century, researchers and clinicians have an opportunity to considerably change the outlook for older adults with ID. Determination of the causes of AD, and effective treatment and prevention of DAD are aspirations which can almost be achieved. Indeed the greatest task faced by the international community will be the satisfactory implementation of future developments worldwide to ensure that all older people with ID benefit from them.

References

Akkerman RL and Ostwald SK (2004) Reducing anxiety in Alzheimer's disease family caregivers: the effectiveness of a nine-week cognitive-behavioral intervention. *Am J Alzheimer Dis Dementias.* **19:** 117–23.

Albert M and Cohen C (1992) The Test for Severe Impairment: an instrument for the assessment of patients with severe cognitive dysfunction. *J Am Geriatr Soc.* **40:** 449–53.

Algase DL (1999) Wandering: a dementia-compromised behavior. *J Gerontol Nurs.* **25:** 10–16.

Alsop D, Kidd M, Landon M and Tomlinson A (1986) Isolated senile plaque cores in Alzheimer's disease and Down's syndrome show differences in morphology. *J Neurol Neurosurg Psychiatry.* **49:** 886–92.

Alzheimer A (1907) Uber eine eigenartige Erkrankung der Hirnrinde. *Alleg Z Psychiatry.* **64:** 146–8.

Amaducci LA, Fratiglioni L, Rocca WA *et al.* (1986) Risk factors for clinically diagnosed Alzheimer's disease: a case–control study of an Italian population. *Neurology.* **36:** 922–31.

American Psychiatric Association (1987) *Diagnostic and Statistical Manual of Mental Disorders, Third Edition Revised.* American Psychiatric Association, Washington, DC.

American Psychiatric Association (1994) *Diagnostic and Statistical Manual of Mental Disorders, Fourth Edition.* American Psychiatric Association, Washington, DC.

Anneren G and Edman B (1993) Down syndrome – a gene dosage disease caused by trisomy of genes within a small segment of the long arm of chromosome 21, exemplified by the study of effects from the superoxide-dismutase type 1 (SOD-1) gene. *APMIS.* **Suppl. 40:** 71–9.

Armstrong RA (1994) Differences in β-amyloid (B/A4) deposition in human patients with Down's syndrome and sporadic Alzheimer's disease. *Neurosci Lett.* **169:** 133–6.

Aylward EH, Burt DB, Thorpe LU and Dalton A (1997) Diagnosis of dementia in individuals with intellectual disability. *J Intellect Disabil Res.* **41:** 152–64.

Azari NP, Pettigrew KD, Pietrini, Horwitz B and Schapiro MB (1994) Detection of an Alzheimer disease pattern of cerebral metabolism in Down syndrome. *Dementia.* **5:** 69–78.

Bachman DL, Wolf PA, Linn RT *et al.* (1993) Incidence of dementia and probable Alzheimer's disease in a general population study: the Framingham Study. *Neurology.* **43:** 515–19.

Baird PA and Sadovnick AD (1989) Life tables for Down syndrome. *Hum Genet.* **82:** 291–2.

Ball MJ and Nuttall K (1980) Neurofibrillary tangles, granulo-vascular degeneration and neuron loss in Down's syndrome: quantitative comparison with Alzheimer's dementia. *Ann Neurol.* **7:** 462–5.

Ballard CG (2002) Advances in the treatment of Alzheimer's disease: benefits of dual cholinesterase inhibition. *Eur Neurol.* **47:** 64–70.

Barcikowska M, Silverman WP, Zigman WB *et al.* (1989) Alzheimer-type neuropathology and clinical symptoms of dementia in mentally retarded people without Down syndrome. *Am J Ment Retard.* **93:** 551–7.

Barry JJ, Lembke A and Bullock KD (2004) Current status of the utilization of antiepileptic treatments in mood, anxiety and aggression: drugs and devices. *Clin EEG Neurosci.* **35:** 4–14.

Bassiony MM, Rosenblatt A, Baker A, Steinberg M, Steele CD and Sheppar Lyketsos CG (2004) Falls and age in patients with Alzheimer's disease. *J Nerv Ment Dis.* **192:** 570–72.

Bates J, Boote J and Beverley C (2004) Psychosocial interventions for people with a milder dementing illness: a systematic review. *J Adv Nurs.* **45:** 644–58.

Berr C, Borghi E, Rethore MO, Lejeune J and Alperovitch A (1989) Absence of familial association between dementia of Alzheimer type and Down syndrome. *Am J Med Genet.* **33**: 545–50.

Bertrand L and Koffas D (1946) Cas d'idiotie mongolienne adulte avec nombreuses plaques seniles et concretions calcaires pallidales. *Rev Neurol (Paris).* **78**: 338–45.

Besson JAO (1994) Magnetic resonance imaging and spectroscopy in dementia. In: A Burns and R Levy (eds) *Dementia.* Chapman & Hall, London.

Blackwood DHR, St Clair DM, Muir WJ, Oliver CJ and Dickens P (1988) The development of Alzheimer's disease in Down's syndrome assessed by auditory event-related potentials. *J Ment Defic Res.* **32**: 439–53.

Bliwise DL (2004) Sleep disorders in Alzheimer's disease and other dementias. *Clin Cornerstone.* **6(1A)**: S16–28.

Blumbergs P, Beran R and Hicks P (1981) Myoclonus in Down's syndrome. *Arch Neurol.* **38**: 453–4.

Bodhireddy S, Dennis W, Mattiace L and Weidenheim KM (1994) A case of Down's syndrome with diffuse Lewy body disease and Alzheimer's disease. *Neurology.* **44**: 159–61.

Braak H and Braak E (1991) Demonstration of amyloid deposits and neurofibrillary changes in whole brain sections. *Brain Pathol.* **1**: 213–16.

Brandel JP, Marconi R, Serdaru M, Vidailhet M and Agid Y (1994) Down's syndrome and Parkinson's disease. *Neurology.* **44**: 2419–20.

Brenner DE, Kukull WA, Stergachis A *et al.* (1994) Postmenopausal estrogen replacement therapy and the risk of Alzheimer's disease: a population-based case–control study. *Am J Epidemiol.* **140**: 262–7.

Brodaty M and Moore CM (1997) The Clock Test for dementia of the Alzheimer's type: a comparison of three scoring methods in a memory disorders clinic. *Int J Geriatr Psychiatry.* **12**: 619–27.

Brodaty H, Howarth GC, Mant A and Kurrle SE (1994) General practice and dementia. A national survey of Australian GPs. *Med J Aust.* **160**: 10–14.

Brugge KL, Nichols SL, Salmon DP *et al.* (1994) Cognitive impairment in adults with Down's syndrome: similarities to early cognitive changes in Alzheimer's disease. *Neurology.* **44**: 232–8.

Burger PC and Vogel FS (1973) The development of the pathologic changes of Alzheimer's disease and senile dementia in patients with Down's syndrome. *Am J Pathol.* **73**: 457–76.

Burns A (1991) Affective symptoms in Alzheimer's disease. *Int J Geriatr Psychiatry.* **6**: 371–6.

Burns A and Pearlson GD (1994) Computed tomography in Alzheimer's disease. In: A Burns and R Levy (eds) *Dementia.* Chapman & Hall, London.

Burns A, Jacoby R, Philpot M and Levy R (1991) CT in Alzheimer's disease – methods of scan analysis, comparison with normal controls and clinical radiological correlations. *Br J Psych.* **159**: 609–14.

Burns A, Philpot M, Costa DC, Ell P and Levy R (1989) Positron emission tomography in dementia: a clinical review. *Int J Geriatr Psychiatry.* **4**: 67–72.

Burns A, Rossor M, Hecker J *et al.* for the International Donepezil Study Group (1999) The effects of donepezil in Alzheimer's disease – results from a multinational trial. *Dementia Geriatr Cogn Disord.* **10**: 237–44.

Burt DB, Loveland KA and Lewis KR (1992) Depression and the onset of dementia in adults with mental retardation. *Am J Ment Retard.* **96**: 502–11.

Buschke H (1973) Selective reminding for analysis of memory and learning. *J Verbal Learn Verbal Behav.* **12**: 543–50.

Buschke H (1984) Cued recall in amnesia. *J Clin Neuropsychol.* **6**: 433–40.

Bush A and Beail N (2004) Risk factors for dementia in people with Down syndrome: issues in assessment and diagnosis. *Am J Ment Retard.* **109**: 83–97.

Cacabelos R, Rodriguez B, Carrera C *et al.* (1996) ApoE-related frequency of cognitive and non-cognitive symptoms in dementia. *Methods Find Exp Clin Pharmacol.* **18**: 693–706.

Cahn DA, Sullivan EV, Shear PK *et al.* (1998) Structural MRI correlates of recognition memory in Alzheimer's disease. *J Int Neuropsychol Soc.* **4**: 106–14.

Cain LF, Levine S and Elzey FF (1963) *Manual for the Cain–Levine Social Competency Scale.* Consulting Psychologists Press, Palo Alto, CA.

Chicoine B and McGuire D (1997) Longevity of a woman with Down syndrome: a case study. *Ment Retard.* **35**: 477–9.

Clark RF and Goate A (1993) Molecular genetics of Alzheimer's disease. *Arch Neurol.* **50**: 1164–72.

Coburn KL, Arruda JE, Estes KM and Amoss RT (2003) Diagnostic utility of visual evoked potential changes in Alzheimer's disease. *J Neuropsychiatry Clin Neurosci.* **15**: 175–9.

Cole G, Neal JW, Singhrao SK, Jasani B and Newman GR (1993) The distribution of amyloid plaques in the cerebellum and brainstem in Down's syndrome and Alzheimer's disease: a light microscopical analysis. *Acta Neuropathol.* **85**: 542–52.

Collman RD and Stoller A (1963) Data on mongolism in Victoria, Australia: prevalence and life expectation. *J Ment Defic Res.* **7**: 60–8.

Cooper S-A (1997a) High prevalence of dementia among people with learning disabilities not attributable to Down's syndrome. *Psychol Med.* **27**: 609–16.

Cooper SA (1997b) A population-based health survey of maladaptive behaviours associated with dementia in elderly people with learning disabilities. *J Intellect Disabil Res.* **41**: 481–7.

Cooper SA and Prasher VP (1998) Maladaptive behaviours and symptoms of dementia in adults with Down's syndrome compared with adults with intellectual disability of other aetiologies. *J Intellect Disabil Res.* **42**: 293–300.

Corder EH, Saunders AM, Strittmatter WJ *et al.* (1993) Gene dose of apolipoprotein E type 4 allele and the risk of Alzheimer's disease in late-onset families. *Science.* **261**: 921–3.

Corder EH, Saunders AM, Strittmatter WJ *et al.* (1995) Apolipoprotein E, survival in Alzheimer's disease patients, and the competing risks of death and Alzheimer's disease. *Neurology.* **45**: 1323–8.

Cosgrave MP, McCarron M, Anderson M, Tyrrell J, Gill M and Lawlor BA (1998) Cognitive decline in Down syndrome: a validity/reliability study of the Test for Severe Impairment. *Am J Ment Retard.* **103**: 193–7.

Cosgrave MP, Tyrrell J, McCarron M, Gill M and Lawlor BA (1999) Age at onset of dementia and age of menopause in women with Down's syndrome. *J Intellect Disabil Res.* **43**: 461–5.

Cosgrave MP, Tyrrell J, McCarron M, Gill M and Lawlor BA (2000) A five-year follow-up study of dementia in persons with Down's syndrome: early symptoms and patterns of deterioration. *Ir J Psychol Med.* **17**: 5–11.

Crapper PR, Dalton AJ, Skopitz, Scott JW and Hachinski VC (1975) Alzheimer degeneration in Down syndrome. *Arch Neurol.* **32**: 618–23.

Cruts M, van Duijn CM and Backhovens H (1998) Estimation of the genetic contribution of presenilin-1 and -2 mutations in a population-based study of presenile Alzheimer disease. *Hum Mol Genet.* **7**: 43–51.

Cuenod CA, Denys A and Michot JL (1993) Amygdala atrophy in Alzheimer's disease. *Arch Neurol.* **50**: 941–5.

Cummings JL, Miller B, Hill MA and Neshkes R (1987) Neuropsychiatric aspects of multi-infarct dementia and dementia of the Alzheimer type. *Arch Neurol.* **44**: 389–93.

Cutler NR (1986) Cerebral metabolism as measured with positron emission tomography (PET) and (^{18}F) 2-deoxy-D-glucose: healthy aging, Alzheimer's disease and Down syndrome. *Prog Neuropsychopharmacol Biol Psychiatry.* **10**: 309–21.

Dalton AJ (1996) *Dyspraxia Scale for Adults with Down Syndrome.* Aging Studies Consortium and Bytecraft Limited, New York.

Dalton AJ and Crapper-McLachlan DR (1984) Incidence of memory deterioration in aging persons with Down's syndrome. In: JM Berg (ed.) *Perspectives and Progress in Mental Retardation: biomedical aspects.* Baltimore University Press, Baltimore, MD.

Dalton AJ and Crapper-McLachlan DR (1986) Clinical expression of Alzheimer's disease in Down's syndrome. *Psychiatr Clin North Am.* **9**: 659–70.

Dalton AJ and Wisniewski HM (1990) Down's syndrome and the dementia of Alzheimer disease. *Int Rev Psychiatry.* **2**: 43–52.

Dalton AJ and McMurray K (1995) *Dalton/McMurray Visual Memory Test.* Aging Studies Consortium and Bytecraft Limited, New York.

Dalton AJ and Fedor BL (1998) Onset of dyspraxia in aging persons with Down syndrome: longitudinal studies. *J Intellect Dev Disabil.* **23**: 13–24.

Dalton AJ, Mehta PD, Fedor BL and Patti PJ (1999) Cognitive changes in memory precede those in praxis in aging persons with Down syndrome. *J Intellect Dev Disabil.* **24**: 169–87.

Dalton AL and Crapper DR (1977) Down's syndrome and ageing of the brain. In: P Mittler (ed.) *Research to Practice in Mental Retardation. Volume 3. Biomedical aspects.* University Park Press, Baltimore, MD.

Dalton AL, Crapper DR and Schlotterer GR (1974) Alzheimer's disease in Down's syndrome: visual retention deficits. *Cortex.* **10**: 366–77.

Dalton AJ, Sano MC, Aisen PS, et al. (2004) Multi-centre Vitamin E trial in ageing persons with Down syndrome. Progress report. *J Intellect Disabil Res.* **48**: 438.

Danysz W, Parsons CG, Mobius HJ, Stoffler A and Quack G (2000) Neuroprotective and symptomatological action of memantine relevant for Alzheimer's disease – a unified hypothesis on the mechanism of action. *Neurotoxicity Res.* **2**: 2–3.

Das JP, Mishra RK, Davison M and Naglieri JA (1995) Measurement of dementia in individuals with mental retardation: comparison based on PPVT and Dementia Rating Scale. *Clin Neuropsychologist.* **9**: 32–7.

Davidson PW, Heller T, Janicki MP and Hyer K (2004) Defining a national health research and practice agenda for older adults with intellectual disabilities. *J Policy Pract Intellect Disabil.* **1**: 2–9.

Day K, Carreon D and Stump C (2000) The therapeutic design of environments for people with dementia: review of the empirical research. *Gerontologist.* **40**: 397–416.

Day KA (1987) The elderly mentally handicapped in hospital: a clinical study. *J Ment Defic Res.* **31**: 131–46.

Deb S and Braganza J (1999) Comparison of rating scales for the diagnosis of dementia in adults with Down's syndrome. *J Intellect Disabil Res.* **43**: 400–7.

Deb S, de Silva PN, Gemmell HG, Beson JAO, Smith FW and Ebmeier KP (1992) Alzheimer's disease in adults with Down's syndrome: the relationship between regional cerebral blood flow equivalents and dementia. *Acta Psychiatr Scand.* **86**: 340–45.

Deb S, Braganza J, Owen M, Kehoe P, Williams H and Norton N (1998) No significant association between a PS-1 intronic polymorphism and dementia in Down's syndrome. *Alzheimer Rep.* **1**: 365–8.

Deb S, Braganza J, Norton N *et al.* (2000) ApoE E4 influences the manifestation of Alzheimer's disease in adults with Down's syndrome. *Br J Psychiatry.* **176**: 468–72.

DeCarli C, Murphy DGM, McIntosh AR, Teichberg D, Schapiro MB and Horwitz B (1995) Discriminant analysis of MRI measures as a method to determine the presence of dementia of the Alzheimer type. *Psychiatry Res.* **57**: 119–30.

Devenny DA, Krinsky-McHale SJ, Sersen G and Silverman WR (2000) Sequence of cognitive decline in dementia in adults with Down's syndrome. *J Intellect Disabil Res.* **44**: 654–65.

Devenny DA, Zimmerli EJ, Kittler P and Krinsky-McHale SJ (2002) Cued recall in early-stage dementia in adults with Down's syndrome. *J Intellect Disabil Res.* **46**: 472–83.

Devinsky O, Sato S, Conmit RA and Schapiro MB (1990) Relation of EEG alpha background to cognitive function, brain atrophy, and cerebral metabolism in Down's syndrome. *Arch Neurol.* **47**: 58–62.

Doody RS, Geldmacher DS, Gordon B, *et al.* (2001) Open-label, multicenter, phase 3 extension study of the safety and efficacy of Donepezil in patients with Alzheimer's disease. *Arch Neurol.* **58:** 427–33.

Dooley M and Lamb HM (2000) Donepezil. A review of its use in Alzheimer's disease. *Drugs Aging.* **3:** 199–226.

Dooley NR and Hinojosa J (2004) Improving quality of life for persons with Alzheimer's disease and their family caregivers: a brief occupational therapy intervention. *Am J Occup Ther.* **58:** 561–9.

Dougall N, Nobili F and Ebmeier KP (2004) Predicting the accuracy of a diagnosis of Alzheimer's disease with 99mTc HMPAO single photon emission computed tomography. *Psychiatry Res.* **131:** 157–68.

Down JL (1862) Observations on an ethnic classification of idiots. *London Hosp Rep.* **3:** 259–62.

Duara R, Barker WW and Lopez-Alberola R (1996) Alzheimer's disease: interaction of apolipoprotein E genotype, family history of dementia, gender, education, ethnicity, and age of onset. *Neurology.* **46:** 1575–9.

Emery VO (2000) Language impairment in dementia of the Alzheimer type: a hierarchical decline? *Int J Psychiatry Med.* **30:** 145–64.

Erkinjuntti T, Lee DH, Gao F *et al.* (1993) Temporal lobe atrophy on magnetic resonance imaging in the diagnosis of early Alzheimer's disease. *Arch Neurol.* **50:** 305–10.

Evenhuis HM (1990) The natural history of dementia in Down's syndrome. *Arch Neurol.* **47:** 263–7.

Evenhuis HM (1992) Evaluation of a screening instrument for dementia in ageing mentally retarded persons. *J Intellect Disabil Res.* **36:** 337–47.

Evenhuis HM (1996) Further evaluation of the Dementia Questionnaire for Persons with Mental Retardation (DMR). *J Intellect Disabil Res.* **40:** 369–73.

Evenhuis HM, Kengen MMF and Eurling HAL (1990) *Dementia Questionnaire for Mentally Retarded Persons.* Hooge Burch, Zwammerdam, The Netherlands.

Eyman RK and Widaman KF (1987) Lifespan development of institutionalised and community-based mentally retarded persons revisited. *Am J Ment Defic.* **91:** 559–69.

Farlow MR (2002) Cholinesterase inhibitors: relating pharmacological properties to clinical profiles. Introduction. *Int J Clin Pract.* **127 (Suppl.):** 1–5.

Farrer MJ, Crayton L, Davies GE *et al.* (1997) Allelic variability in D21S11, but not in APP or ApoE, is associated with cognitive decline in Down syndrome. *Neuroreport.* **8:** 1645–9.

Fenner ME, Hewitt KE and Torpy M (1987) Down's syndrome: intellectual and behavioural functioning during adulthood. *J Ment Defic Res.* **31:** 241–9.

Folstein ME, Folstein SE and McHugh PR (1975) Mini-Mental State: a practical method for grading the cognitive state of patients for the clinician. *J Psychiatr Res.* **12:** 189–98.

Forster DP, Newens AJ, Kay DW, *et al.* (1995) Risk factors in clinically diagnosed presenile dementia of the Alzheimer type: a case–control study in northern England. *J Epidemiol Community Health.* **49:** 253–8.

Frangou S, Aylward E, Warren A, Sharma T, Barta P and Pearlson G (1997) Small planum temporale volume in Down's syndrome: a volumetric MRI study. *Am J Psychiatry.* **154:** 1424–9.

Fraser J and Mitchell A (1876) Kalmuc idiocy: report of a case with autopsy with notes on 62 cases. *J Ment Sci.* **22:** 161.

Fratiglioni L, Grut M, Forsell Y *et al.* (1991) Prevalence of Alzheimer's disease and other dementias in an elderly urban population: relationship with age, sex and education. *Neurology.* **41:** 1886–92.

Galasko D, Hansen LA, Katzman R *et al.* (1994) Clinical–neuropathological correlations in Alzheimer's disease and related dementias. *Arch Neurol.* **51:** 888–95.

Games D, Adams D, Alessandrini R *et al.* (1995) Alzheimer-type neuropathology in transgenic mice overexpressing V717f beta-amyloid precurosor protein. *Nature.* **373:** 523–7.

Gedye A (1991) Serotonergic treatment for aggression in a Down's syndrome adult showing signs of Alzheimer's disease. *J Ment Defic Res.* **35:** 247–58.

Gedye A (1995) *Dementia Scale for Down Syndrome: manual.* Gedye Research & Consulting, Vancouver.

Geldmacher DS, Lerner AJ, Voci JM, Noelker EA, Somple LC and Whitehouse PJ (1997) Treatment of functional decline in adults with Down syndrome: selective serotonin reuptake inhibitor drugs. *J Geriatr Psychiatry Neurol.* **10:** 99–104.

Gertz HJ and Kiefer M (2004) Review about *Ginkgo biloba* special extract EGb 761 (*Ginkgo*). *Curr Pharm Design.* **10:** 261–4.

Gill SS, Rochon PA, Herrmann N *et al.* (2005) Atypical antipsychotic drugs and risk of ischaemic stroke: population-based retrospective cohort study. *BMJ.* **330:** 445–8.

Glenner GG and Wong CW (1984) Alzheimer's disease: initial report of the purification and characterization of a novel cerebrovascular amyloid protein. *Biochem Biophys Res Commun.* **120:** 885–90.

Goate AM, Chartier-Harlene CM and Mullan M (1991) Segregation of a missense mutation in the amyloid precursor protein gene with familial Alzheimer's disease. *Nature.* **353:** 844–6.

Gomez-Isla T, West HL, Rebeck GW *et al.* (1996) Clinical and pathological correlates of apolipoprotein E4 in Alzheimer's disease. *Ann Neurol.* **39:** 62–70.

Good DC and Howard HD (1982) Myoclonus in Down's syndrome: treatment with clonazepam. *Arch Neurol.* **39:** 195.

Goodman C (1986) Research on the informal carer: a selected literature review. *J Adv Nurs.* **11:** 705–12.

Granholm AC, Sanders L, Seo H, Lin L, Ford K and Isacson O (2003) Estrogen alters amyloid precursor protein as well as dendritic and cholinergic markers in a mouse model of Down syndrome. *Hippocampus.* **13:** 905–14.

Growdon JH, Locascio JJ, Corkin S, Gomez-Isla T and Hyman BT (1996) Apolipoprotein E genotype does not influence rates of cognitive decline in Alzheimer's disease. *Neurology.* **47:** 444–8.

Hachinski VC, Iliff LD, Zilhka E *et al.* (1975) Cerebral blood flow in dementia. *Arch Neurol.* **32:** 632–7.

Haier RJ, Alkire MT, White NS *et al.* (2003) Temporal cortex hypermetabolism in Down syndrome prior to the onset of dementia. *Neurology.* **61:** 1673–9.

Hardy J, Crook R, Perry R, Raghavan R and Roberts G (1994) ApoE genotype and Down's syndrome. *Lancet.* **343:** 979–80.

Harvey GT, Hughes J, McKeith IG *et al.* (1999) Magnetic resonance imaging differences between dementia with Lewy bodies and Alzheimer's disease: a pilot study. *Psychol Med.* **29:** 181–7.

Haxby JV (1989) Neuropsychological evaluation of adults with Down's syndrome: patterns of selective impairment in non-demented old adults. *J Ment Defic Res.* **33:** 193–210.

Head E and Lott IT (2004) Down syndrome and beta-amyloid deposition. *Curr Opin Neurol.* **17:** 95–100.

Henderson JG, Strachan RW, Beck JS, Dawson AA and Daniel M (1966) The antigastric-antibody test as a screening procedure for vitamin B_{12} deficiency in psychiatric practice. *Lancet.* **2:** 809–13.

Henderson VW, Paganini-Hill A, Miller BL *et al.* (2000) Estrogen for Alzheimer's disease in women: randomized, double-blind, placebo-controlled trial. *Neurology.* **54:** 295–301.

Hendriks L and van Broeckhoven C (1996) The beta A4 amyloid precursor protein gene and Alzheimer's disease. *Eur J Biochem.* **237:** 6–15.

Hesdorffer DC, Hauser WA, Annegers JF, Kokmen E and Rocca WA (1996) Dementia and adult-onset unprovoked seizures. *Neurology.* **46:** 727–30.

Heston LL, Mastri AR, Anderson VE and White J (1981) Dementia of the Alzheimer type. Clinical genetics, natural history and associated conditions. *Arch Gen Psychiatry.* **38:** 1085–90.

Hewitt KE, Carter G and Jancer J (1985) Ageing in Down's syndrome. *Br J Psychiatry.* **147:** 58–62.

Heyman A, Wilkinson WE, Stafford JA, Helma MJ, Sigmon AH and Weinberg T (1984) Alzheimer's disease: a study of epidemiological aspects. *Ann Neurol.* **15:** 335–41.

Hof PR, Perl DP, Sparks L, Mehta N and Morrison JH (1995) Age-related distribution of neuropathologic changes in the cerebral cortex of patients with Down's syndrome. *Arch Neurol.* **52:** 379–91.

Hofman A, Rocca WA, Brayne C, Breteler M, Clarke M and Cooper B (1991) The prevalence of dementia in Europe: a collaborative study of 1980–1990 findings. *Int J Epidemiol.* **20:** 736–48.

Holland AJ, Hon J, Huppert FA, Stevens F and Watson P (1998) Population-based study of the prevalence and presentation of dementia in adults with Down's syndrome. *Br J Psychiatry.* **172:** 493–8.

Holland AJ, Hon J, Huppert FA and Stevens F (2000) Incidence and course of dementia in people with Down's syndrome: findings from a population-based study. *J Intellect Disabil Res.* **44:** 138–46.

Horwitz, B, Schapiro MB, Grady CL and Rapport SI (1990) Cerebral metabolic pattern in young adult Down's syndrome subjects: altered intercorrelations between regional rates of glucose utilization. *J Ment Defic Res.* **34:** 237–52.

Huff FJ, Auerbach J, Chakravarti A and Boller F (1988) Risk of dementia in relatives of patients with Alzheimer's disease. *Neurology.* **38:** 786–90.

Hughes CP, Berg L, Danziger WL, Coben LA and Martin RL (1982) A new clinical scale for the staging of dementia. *Br J Psychiatry.* **140:** 566–72.

Hutchinson NJ (1999) Association between Down's syndrome and Alzheimer's disease: review of the literature. *J Learn Disabil Nurs Health Soc Care.* **3:** 194–203.

Huxley A, Prasher VP and Haque MS (2000) The dementia scale for Down's syndrome. *J Intellect Disabil Res.* **44:** 697–8.

Ikeda M and Arai Y (2002) Longitudinal changes in brain CT scans and development of dementia in Down's syndrome. *Eur Neurol.* **47:** 205–8.

Imbimbo BP (2004) The potential role of non-steroidal anti-inflammatory drugs in treating Alzheimer's disease. *Expert Opin Invest Drugs.* **13:** 1469–81.

Insau P and Lawley D (2004) CSM guidance on antipsychotic use in care of the elderly. *Geriatr Med.* **July:** 6–7.

Iwatsubo T, Odaka A, Suzuki N *et al.* (1994) Visualization of AB42 (43) and AB40 in senile plaques with end-specific AB monoclonals: evidence that an initially deposited species is AB42 (43). *Neuron.* **13:** 45–53.

Jacobson JW and Janicki MP (1985) Clinical need variations of disabled persons residing in group homes. *J Commun Psychol.* **13:** 54–66.

Janicki MP and Jacobson JW (1986) Generational trends in sensory, physical and behavioural abilities among older mentally retarded persons. *Am J Ment Defic.* **90:** 490–500.

Janicki MP and Dalton AJ (2000) Prevalence of dementia and impact on intellectual disability services. *Ment Retard.* **38:** 276–88.

Janicki MP, Heller T, Seltzer GB and Hogg J (1996) Practice guidelines for the clinical assessment and care management of Alzheimer's disease and other dementias among adults with intellectual disability. *J Intellect Disabil Res.* **40:** 374–82.

Jarvik LF, Ruth V and Matsuyama SS (1980) Organic brain syndrome and aging. A six-year follow-up of surviving twins. *Arch Gen Psychiatry.* **37:** 280–6.

Jeong J (2004) EEG dynamics in patients with Alzheimer's disease. *Clin Neurophysiol.* **115:** 1490–505.

Jernigan TL, Butters N and Hesselink JR (1991) Cerebral structure on MRI. Part II. Specific changes in Alzheimer's and Huntington's diseases. *Biol Psychiatry.* **29:** 68–81.

Jervis GA (1948) Early senile dementia mongoloid idiocy. *Am J Psychiatry.* **105:** 102–6.

Johanson A, Gustafson L, Brun A, Risberg J, Rosen I. and Tideman E (1991) A longitudinal study of dementia of Alzheimer type in Down's syndrome. *Dementia.* **2:** 159–68.

Jones AM, Kennedy N, Hanson J and Fenton GW (1997) A study of dementia in adults with Down's syndrome using 99Tcm-HMPAO SPECT. *Nucl Med Commun.* **18:** 662–7.

Kalia M (2003) Dysphagia and aspiration pneumonia in patients with Alzheimer's disease. *Metabolism.* **52:** 36–8.

Kanai M, Shizuka M, Urakami K *et al.* (1999) Apolipoprotein E4 accelerates dementia and increases cerebrospinal fluid tau levels in Alzheimer's disease. *Neurosci Lett.* **267:** 65–8.

Kang J, Lemaire HG, Unterbeck A *et al.* (1987) The precursor of Alzheimer's disease, amyloid A4 protein, resembles a cell surface receptor. *Nature.* **325:** 733–6.

Kao CH, Wang PY, Wang SJ *et al.* (1993) Regional cerebral blood flow of Alzheimer's disease-like pattern in young patients with Down's syndrome detected by [99]Tcm-HMPAO SPECT. *Nucl Med Commun.* **14:** 47–51.

Kertesz A, Polk M and Carr T (1990) Cognition and white matter changes on magnetic resonance imaging in dementia. *Arch Neurol.* **47:** 387–91.

Kesslak JP, Nagata SF, Lott I and Nalcioglu O (1994) Magnetic resonance imaging analysis of age-related changes in the brains of individuals with Down's syndrome. *Neurology.* **44:** 1039–45.

Killiany RJ, Moss MB, Albert MS, Sandor T, Tieman J and Jolesz F (1993) Temporal lobe regions on magnetic resonance imaging identify patients with early Alzheimer's disease. *Arch Neurol.* **50:** 949–54.

Kishnani PS, Sullivan JA, Walter BK, Spiridigliozzi GA, Doraiswamy PM and Krishnan KRR (1999) Cholinergic therapy for Down's syndrome. *Lancet.* **353:** 1064–6.

Kledaras JB, McIlvane WJ and Mackay HA (1989) Progressive decline of picture naming in an aging Down syndrome man with dementia. *Percept Mot Skills.* **69:** 1091–100.

Knott V, Mohr E, Mahoney C and Ilivitsky V (2000) Electroencephalographic coherence in Alzheimer's disease: comparisons with a control group and population norms. *J Geriatr Psychiatry Neurol.* **13:** 1–8.

Kral VA (1962) Senescent forgetfulness: benign and malignant. *Can Med Assoc J.* **86:** 257–60.

Krinsky-McHale SJ, Devenny DA and Silverman WP (2002) Changes in explicit memory associated with early dementia in adults with Down's syndrome. *J Intellect Disabil Res.* **46:** 198–208.

Kukull WA, Schellenberg GD, Bowen JD *et al.* (1996) Apolipoprotein E in Alzheimer's disease risk and case detection: a case–control study. *J Clin Epidemiol.* **49:** 1143–8.

Laakso MP, Soininen H, Partanen K *et al.* (1995) Volumes of hippocampus, amygdala and frontal lobes in the MRI-based diagnosis of early Alzheimer's disease: correlation with memory functions. *J Neural Transm.* **9:** 73–86.

Lai F and Williams RS (1989) A prospective study of Alzheimer disease in Down syndrome. *Arch Neurol.* **46:** 849–53.

Lai F, Kammann E, Rebeck GW, Anderson A, Chen Y and Nixon RA (1999) ApoE genotype and gender effects on Alzheimer disease in 100 adults with Down syndrome. *Neurology.* **53:** 331–6.

Lambert J-C, Perez-Tur J, Dupire M-J, Delacourte A, Frigard B and Chartier-Harlin M-C (1996) Analysis of the ApoE alleles: impact in Down's syndrome. *Neurosci Lett.* **200:** 57–60.

Lawlor BA (2004) Behavioral and psychological symptoms in dementia: the role of atypical antipsychotics. *J Clin Psychiatry.* **65:** 5–10.

Lawlor BA, McCarron M, Wilson G and McLoughlin M (2001) Temporal lobe-orientated CT scanning and dementia in Down's syndrome. *Int J Geriatr Psychiatry.* **16:** 427–9.

Lejeune L, Gautier M and Turpin R (1959) Les chromosomes humains en culture de tisshu. *Comptes Rendus Acad Sci.* **248:** 602–3.

LeMay M and Alvarez N (1990) The relationship between enlargement of the temporal horns of the lateral ventricles and dementia in aging patients with Down syndrome. *Neuroradiology.* **32:** 104–7.

Lehtovirta M, Soininen H, Laakso MP *et al.* (1996) SPECT and MRI analysis in Alzheimer's disease: relation to apolipoprotein E epsilon 4 allele. *J Neurol Neurosurg Psychiatry.* **60:** 644–9.

Lendon CL, Talbot CJ, Craddock NJ *et al.* (1997) Genetic association studies between dementia of the Alzheimer's type and three receptors for apolipoprotein E in a Caucasian population. *Neurosci Lett.* **222:** 187–90.

Levy R (1994) Aging-associated cognitive decline. *Int Psychogeriatr.* **6:** 63–8.

Levy-Lahad E, Tsuang D and Bird TD (1998) Recent advances in the genetics of Alzheimer's disease. *J Geriatr Psychiatry Neurol.* **11:** 42–54.

Liddell M, Williams J, Bayer A, Kaiser F and Owen M (1994) Confirmation of association between the e4 allele of apolipoprotein E and Alzheimer's disease. *J Med Genet.* **31:** 197–200.

Liss L, Shim C, Thase M, Smeltzer D, Maloone J and Couri D (1980) The relationship between Down's syndrome and dementia of Alzheimer's type. *J Neuropathol Exp Neurol.* **39:** 371.

Lorenzo-Otero J (2001) Apraxia of ideas and movements and visual-constructive skills. *Rev Neurol.* **32:** 473–7.

Lott IT and Lai F (1982) Dementia in Down syndrome: observations from a neurology clinic. *Appl Res Ment Defic.* **3:** 223–39.

Lott IT, Osann K, Doran E and Nelson L (2002) Down syndrome and Alzheimer disease: response to donepezil. *Arch Neurol.* **59:** 1133–6.

Lyketsos CG and Lee HB (2004) Diagnosis and treatment of depression in Alzheimer's disease. A practical update for the clinician. *Dementia Geriatr Cogn Disord.* **17:** 55–64.

McCarron M (1999) Some issues in caring for people with the dual disability of Down's syndrome and Alzheimer's dementia. *J Learn Disabil.* **3:** 123–9.

McCarron M, Gill M, Lawlor B and Begley C (2002) Time spent caregiving for persons with the dual disability of Down's syndrome and Alzheimer's dementia. *J Learn Disabil.* **6:** 263–79.

McCarthy JM and Mullan E (1996) The elderly with a learning disability (mental retardation): an overview. *Int Psychogeriatr.* **8:** 489–501.

McDonald WM, Ranga K, Krishnan R *et al.* (1991) Magnetic resonance findings in patients with early-onset Alzheimer's disease. *Biol Psychiatry.* **29:** 799–810.

McGeer PL and McGeer EG (1996) Anti-inflammatory drugs in the fight against Alzheimer's disease. *Ann N Y Acad Sci.* **17:** 213–20.

McGeer PL and McGeer EG (1998) Mechanisms of cell death in Alzheimer disease: immunopathology. *J Neural Transm.* **54:** 159–66.

McGonigal G, Thomas B, McQuade C, Starr JM, MacLennan WJ and Whalley LJ (1993) Epidemiology of Alzheimer's presenile dementia in Scotland, 1974–88. *BMJ.* **306:** 680–83.

McKann G, Drachman D, Folstein M, Katzman R, Price D and Stadlan EM (1984) Clinical diagnosis of Alzheimer's disease: report of the NINCDS–ADRDA Work Group under the auspices of the Department of Health and Human Services Task Force on Alzheimer's Disease. *Neurology.* **34:** 939–44.

Malamud N (1966) The neuropathology of mental retardation. In: I Phillips (ed.) *Prevention and Treatment of Mental Retardation.* Basic Books, New York.

Mangone CA (2004) Clinical heterogeneity of Alzheimer's disease. Different clinical profiles can predict the progression rate. *Rev Neurol.* **38:** 675–81.

Mann DMA (1988) The pathological association between Down syndrome and Alzheimer disease. *Mech Ageing Dev.* **43:** 99–136.

Mann DMA, Pickering-Brown SM, Siddons MA *et al.* (1995) The extent of amyloid deposition in brain in patients with Down's syndrome does not depend upon the apolipoprotein E genotype. *Neurosci Lett.* **196:** 105–8.

Margallo-Lana ML, Ballard C, Morris C, Kay D, Tyrer S and Moore B (2003) Cholinesterase inhibitors in the treatment of dementia. *Int J Geriatr Psychiatry.* **18:** 458–9.

Margallo-Lana M, Morris CM, Gibson AM *et al.* (2004) Influence of the amyloid precursor protein locus on dementia in Down syndrome. *Neurology.* **62**: 1996–8.

Marriott A, Donaldson C, Tarrier N and Burns A (2000) Effectiveness of cognitive-behavioural family intervention in reducing the burden of care in carers of patients with Alzheimer disease. *Br J Psychiatry.* **178**: 83–4.

Martin A (2003) Antioxidant vitamins E and C and risk of Alzheimer's disease. *Nutr Rev.* **61**: 69–73.

Martin RL, Gerteis G and Gabrielli WF Jr (1988) A family genetic study of dementia of Alzheimer type. *Arch Gen Psychiatry.* **45**: 894–900.

Martins RN, Clarnette R, Fisher C *et al.* (1995) ApoE genotypes in Australia: roles in early and late onset Alzheimer's disease and Down's syndrome. *Neuroreport.* **6**: 1513–16.

Maruyama K, Ikeda S and Yanagisawa N (1995) Correlative study of the brain CT and clinical features of patients with Down's syndrome in three clinical stages of Alzheimer-type dementia. *Rinsho Shinkeigaku.* **35**: 775–80.

Matsuda H (2001) Cerebral blood flow and metabolic abnormalities in Alzheimer's disease. *Ann Nucl Med.* **15**: 85–92.

Mayeux R, Saunders A, Shea S *et al.* (1998) Utility of the apolipoprotein E genotype in the diagnosis of Alzheimer's disease. *NEJM.* **338**: 506–11.

Mehta PD, Dalton AJ, Mehta SP, Soo Kim K, Sersen EA and Wisniewski HM (1998) Increased plasma amyloid β protein 1–42 levels in Down syndrome. *Neurosci Lett.* **241**: 13–16.

Melamed E, Mildworf B, Sharav T, Belenky L and Wertman E (1987) Regional cerebral blood flow in Down's syndrome. *Ann Neurol.* **22**: 275–8.

Mendez MF, Mendez MA, Martin R, Smyth KA and Whitehouse PJ (1990) Complex visual disturbances in Alzheimer's disease. *Neurology.* **40**: 439–43.

Mendez MF, Catanzaro P, Doss RC, Arguello R and Frey WH II (1994) Seizures in Alzheimer's disease: clinico-pathologic study. *J Geriatr Psychiatry Neurol.* **7**: 230–3.

Mielke R and Heiss WD (1998) Positron emission tomography for diagnosis of Alzheimer's disease and vascular dementia. *J Neural Transm.* **53 (Suppl.)**: 237–50.

Mittelman MS, Ferris SH, Shulman E *et al.* (1996) A family intervention to delay nursing home placement of patients with Alzheimer's disease. A randomized controlled trial. *J Am Med Assoc.* **276**: 1725–31.

Mohs RC, Doody RS, Morris JC *et al.* (2001) A 1-year, placebo-controlled preservation of function survival study of Donepezil in AD patients. *Neurol.* **57**: 481–8.

Moller JC, Hamer HM, Oertel WH and Rosenow F (2001) Late-onset myoclonic epilepsy in Down's syndrome (LOMEDS). *Seizure.* **10**: 303–5.

Moore NC (1997) Visual evoked responses in Alzheimer's disease: a review. *Clin Electro-encephalogr.* **28**: 137–42.

Morris JC, Heyman A, Mohs RC *et al.* (1989) The Consortium to Establish a Registry for Alzheimer's Disease (CERAD). Part I. Clinical and neuropsychological assessment of Alzheimer's disease. *Neurology.* **39**: 1159–65.

Mortimer JA, van Duijn CM, Chandra V *et al.* (1991) Head trauma as a risk factor for Alzheimer's disease: a collaborative re-analysis of case–control studies. EURODEM Risk Factors Research Group. *Int J Epidemiol.* **20 (Suppl. 2)**: S28–35.

Moss S and Patel P (1995) Psychiatric symptoms associated with dementia in older people with learning disability. *Br J Psychiatry.* **167**: 663–7.

Moss SC, Patel P, Prosser H *et al.* (1993) Psychiatric morbidity in older people with moderate and severe learning disability (mental retardation). Part I. Development and reliability of the patient interview (the PAS-ADD). *Br J Psychiatry.* **163**: 471–80.

Motonaga K, Itoh M, Becker LE, Goto Y and Takashima S (2002) Elevated expression of beta-site amyloid precursor protein cleaving enzyme 2 in brains of patients with Down syndrome. *Neurosci Lett.* **326**: 64–6.

Motte J and Williams RS (1989) Age-related changes in the density and morphology of plaques and neurofibrillary tangles in Down syndrome brain. *Acta Neuropathol.* **77**: 535–46.

Muir WJ, Squire I, Blackwood DHR *et al.* (1988) Auditory P300 response in the assessment of Alzheimer's disease in Down's syndrome: a 2-year follow-up study. *J Ment Defic Res.* **32:** 455–63.

Murphy GM, Taylor J, Kraemer HC, Yesavage J and Tinklenberg JR (1997) No association between apolipoprotein E4 allele and rate of decline in Alzheimer's disease. *Am J Psychiatry.* **154:** 603–8.

Nakamura H (1961) Nature of institutionalised adult mongoloid intelligence. *Am J Ment Defic.* **66:** 456–8.

National Institute for Clinical Excellence (2001) *Guidance on the Use of Donepezil, Rivastigmine and Galantamine for the Treatment of Alzheimer's Disease.* National Institute for Clinical Excellence, London.

O'Brien JT, Ames D, Schweitzer I, Colman P, Desmond P and Tress B (1996) Clinical and magnetic resonance imaging correlates of hypothalamic–pituitary–adrenal axis function in depression and Alzheimer's disease. *Br J Psychiatry.* **168:** 679–87.

Ojemann RG (1971) Normal pressure hydrocephalus. *Clin Neurosurg.* **18:** 337–70.

Olichney JM and Hillert DG (2004) Clinical applications of cognitive event-related potentials in Alzheimer's disease. *Phys Med Rehabil Clin North Am.* **15:** 205–33.

Oliver C and Holland AJ (1986) Down's syndrome and Alzheimer's disease: a review. *Psychol Med.* **16:** 307–22.

Oliver C, Crayton L, Holland A and Hall S (2000) Cognitive deterioration in adults with Down syndrome: effects on the individual, caregivers, and service use. *Am J Ment Retard.* **105:** 455–65.

Owens D, Dawson JC and Losin S (1971) Alzheimer's disease in Down's syndrome. *Am J Ment Defic.* **75:** 606–12.

Pantel J, Schroder J, Schad LR *et al.* (1997) Quantitative magnetic resonance imaging and neuropsychological functions in dementia of the Alzheimer type. *Psychol Med.* **27:** 221–9.

Patel P, Goldberg D and Moss S (1993) Psychiatric morbidity in older people with moderate and severe learning disabilities. II. The prevalence study. *Br J Psychiatry.* **163:** 481–91.

Pearlson GD, Ross CA, Lohr WD, Rovner BW, Chase GA and Folstein MF (1990) Association between family history of affective disorder and the depressive syndrome of Alzheimer's disease. *Am J Psychiatry.* **147:** 452–6.

Pearlson GD, Breiter SN, Aylward EH *et al.* (1998) MRI brain changes in subjects with Down syndrome with and without dementia. *Dev Med Child Neurol.* **40:** 326–34.

Pelz DM, Karlik SJ, Fox AJ and Vinuela F (1986) Magnetic resonance imaging in Down's syndrome. *Can J Neurol Sci.* **13:** 566–9.

Penrose LS (1949) The incidence of mongolism in the general population. *J Ment Sci.* **95:** 685.

Perl DP (2000) Neuropathology of Alzheimer's disease and related disorders. *Neurol Clin.* **18:** 847–64.

Pietrini P, Dani A, Furey ML *et al.* (1997) Low glucose metabolism during brain stimulation in older Down's syndrome subjects at risk for Alzheimer's disease prior to dementia. *Am J Psychiatry.* **154:** 1063–9.

Pintiaux A, Van den Brule F, Foidart JM and Gaspard U (2003) Hormone replacement therapy one year after the results of the Women's Health Initiative. *Rev Med Liege.* **58:** 572–5.

Pitkanen A, Laakso M, Kalviainen R *et al.* (1996) Severity of hippocampal atrophy correlates with the prolongation of MRI T2 relaxation time in temporal lobe epilepsy but not in Alzheimer's disease. *Neurology.* **46:** 1724–30.

Poirier J, Danik M and Blass JP (1999) Pathophysiology of the Alzheimer syndrome. In: S Gauthier (ed.) *Clinical Diagnosis and Management of Alzheimer's Disease.* Martin Dunitz, London.

Politoff AL, Stadter RP, Monson N and Hass P (1996) Cognition-related EEG abnormalities in non-demented Down syndrome subjects. *Dementia.* **7:** 69–75.

Popovitch ER, Wisniewski HM, Barcikowska M *et al.* (1990) Alzheimer neuropathology in non-Down's syndrome mentally retarded adults. *Acta Neuropathol.* **80:** 362–7.

Poulin P and Zakzanis KK (2002) *In vivo* neuroanatomy of Alzheimer's disease: evidence from structural and functional brain imaging. *Brain Cogn.* **49:** 220–25.

Prasher VP (1993) Presenile dementia associated with unbalanced Robertsonian translocation form of Down's syndrome. *Lancet.* **342:** 686–7.

Prasher VP (1994) Temporal relationship between clinical and neuropathological dementia in people with Down syndrome. *Br J Clin Soc Psychiatry.* **9:** 24–5.

Prasher VP (1995a) Age-specific prevalence, thyroid dysfunction and depressive symptomatology in adults with Down syndrome and dementia. *Int J Geriatr Psychiatry.* **10:** 25–31.

Prasher V (1995b) End-stage dementia in adults with Down syndrome. *Int J Geriatr Psychiatry.* **10:** 1067–9.

Prasher VP (1996) Presenile dementia in a Down syndrome adult with an unbalanced 21/ 21 Robertsonian translocation. *Br J Psychiatry.* **168:** 521–2.

Prasher VP (1997a) Psychotic features and effect on severity of learning disability on dementia in adults with Down syndrome. Review of literature. *Br J Develop Dis.* **43:** 85–92.

Prasher VP (1997b) Dementia questionnaire for persons with mental retardation (DMR). Modified criteria for adults with Down syndrome. *J Appl Res Intellect Dis.* **10:** 54–60.

Prasher V (1998) Adaptive behavior. In: MP Janicki and AJ Dalton (eds) *Dementia, Aging and Intellectual Disabilities.* Taylor & Francis, Philadelphia, PA.

Prasher VP (1999) Down syndrome and thyroid disorders: a review. *Down Syndr Res Pract.* **6:** 105–10.

Prasher VP (2003) The role of donepezil in the treatment of dementia in Alzheimer's disease in adults with Down syndrome. In: A Malard (ed.) *Focus on Down Syndrome.* Nova Biomedical Books, NY.

Prasher VP (2004) Review of donepezil, rivastigmine, galantamine and memantine for the treatment of dementia in AD in adults with Down syndrome: implications for the intellectual disability population. *Int J Geriatr Psychiatry.* **19:** 1–7.

Prasher VP and Corbett JA (1993) Onset of seizures as a poor indicator of longevity in people with Down syndrome and dementia. *Int J Geriatr Psychiatry.* **8:** 1–5.

Prasher VP and Krishnan VHR (1993) Age of onset and duration of dementia in people with Down syndrome: integration of 98 reported cases in the literature. *Int J Geriatr Psychiatry.* **8:** 915–22.

Prasher VP and Filer A (1995) Behavioural disturbance in people with Down's syndrome and dementia. *J Intellect Disabil Res.* **39:** 432–6.

Prasher VP and Blair JA (1996) Low blood pressure and dementia in elderly people. *BMJ.* **313:** 111.

Prasher VP and Hall W (1996) Short-term prognosis of depression in adults with Down syndrome: association with thyroid status and effects on adaptive behaviour. *J Intellect Disabil Res.* **40:** 32–8.

Prasher VP, Krishnan VHR, Clarke DJ, Corbett JA and Blake A (1994) Visual evoked potential in the diagnosis of dementia in people with Down syndrome. *Int J Geriatr Psychiatry.* **9:** 473–8.

Prasher VP, Chowdhury TA, Rowe BR and Bain SC (1997) ApoE genotype and Alzheimer's disease in adults with Down syndrome: meta-analysis. *Am J Ment Retard.* **102:** 103–10.

Prasher VP, Farrer MJ, Kessling AM *et al.* (1998) Molecular mapping of Alzheimer-type dementia in Down syndrome. *Ann Neurol.* **43:** 380–83.

Prasher VP, Viswanathan J and Holder R (2002a) Down syndrome, dementia and macrocytosis. *Ir J Psychol Med.* **19:** 115–20.

Prasher VP, Huxley A and Haque S (2002b) A 24-week, double-blind, placebo-controlled trial of donepezil in patients with Down syndrome and Alzheimer's disease: pilot study. *Int J Geriatr Psychiatry.* **17:** 270–78.

Prasher VP, Adams C and Holder R (2003a) Long-term safety and efficacy of donepezil in the treatment of dementia in Alzheimer's disease in adults with Down syndrome: open-label study. *Int J Geriatr Psychiatry.* **8:** 549–51.

Prasher V, Cumella S, Natarajan K, Rolfe E, Shah S and Haque S (2003b) Magnetic resonance imaging, Down's syndrome and Alzheimer's disease: research and clinical implications. *J Intellect Disabil Res.* **47:** 90–100.

Prasher VP, Metseagharun T and Haque S (2004) Weight loss in adults with Down syndrome and with dementia in Alzheimer's disease. *Res Dev Disabil.* **25:** 1–7.

Prasher VP, Fung N and Adams C (2005) Rivastigmine in the treatment of dementia in Alzheimer's disease in adults with Down syndrome. *Int J Geriatr Psychiatry.* **20:** 496–7.

Puri BK, Zhang Z and Singh I (1994) SPECT in adult mosaic Down's syndrome with early dementia. *Clin Nucl Med.* **19:** 989–91.

Qureshi K and Hodkinson M (1974) Evaluation of a 10-question mental test of the institutionalised elderly. *Age Ageing.* **3:** 152–7.

Rae-Grant AD, Barbour PJ, Sirotta P and Gross P (1991) Alzheimer's disease in Down's syndrome with SPECT. *Clin Nucl Med.* **16:** 509–10.

Raghavan R, Khin-Nu C, Brown A *et al.* (1993) Detection of Lewy bodies in trisomy 21 (Down's syndrome). *Can J Neurol Sci.* **20:** 48–51.

Raghavan R, Khin-Nu C, Brown AG *et al.* (1994) Gender differences in the phenotypic expression of Alzheimer's disease in Down's syndrome (trisomy 21). *Neuroreport.* **5:** 1393–6.

Raz N, Torres IJ, Briggs SD *et al.* (1995) Selective neuroanatomic abnormalities in Down's syndrome and their cognitive correlates: evidence from MRI morphometry. *Neurology.* **45:** 356–66.

Reisberg B, Ferris SH, de Leon MJ and Crook T (1988) Global Deterioration Scale (GDS). *Psychopharmacol Bull.* **24:** 661–3.

Robakis NK, Wisniewski HM, Jenkins EC, Devine-Gage EA, Houck GE and Yao XL (1987) Chromosome 21q21 sublocalization of gene encoding beta-amyloid peptide in cerebral vessels and neuritic (senile) plaques of people with Alzheimer's disease and Down's syndrome. *Lancet.* **1:** 384–5.

Robinson KC, Kallberg MH and Crowley MF (1954) Idiopathic hypoparathyroidism presenting as dementia. *BMJ.* **4898:** 1203–6.

Rollin HR (1946) Personality in mongolism, with special reference to catatonic psychosis. *Am J Ment Defic.* **51:** 219–37.

Ropper AH and Williams RS (1980) Relationship between plaques, tangles and dementia in Down's syndrome. *Neurology.* **30:** 639–44.

Roses AD (1994) Apolipoprotein E affects the rate of Alzheimer disease expression: beta-amyloid burden is a secondary consequence dependent on ApoE genotype and duration of disease. *J Neuropathol Exp Neurol.* **53:** 429–37.

Rossi R, Joachim C, Smith AD and Frisoni GB (2004) The CT-based radial width of the temporal horn: pathological validation in AD without cerebrovascular disease. *Int J Geriatr Psychiatry.* **19:** 570–74.

Roth GM, Sun B, Greensite FS, Lott IT and Dietrich RB (1996) Premature aging in persons with Down syndrome: MR findings. *Am J Neuroradiol.* **17:** 1283–9.

Roth M, Tym E, Mounyjoy *et al.* (1986) CAMDEX. A standardised instrument for the diagnosis of mental disorder in the elderly with special reference to the early detection of dementia. *Br J Psychiatry.* **149:** 698–709.

Rowe IF, Ridler MAC and Gibberd FB (1989) Presenile dementia associated with mosaic trisomy 21 in a patient with Down syndrome. *Lancet.* **ii:** 229.

Royal College of Psychiatrists (2004) *Atypical Antipsychotics and BPSD. Summary of prescribing update for old age psychiatrists.* Atypical Antipsychotic Prescribing Update Summary. Royal College of Psychiatrists, London.

Royston MC, Mann D, Pickering-Brown OF *et al.* (1994) Apolipoprotein E ε2 allele promotes longevity and protects patients with Down syndrome from dementia. *Neuroreport.* **5:** 2583–5.

Rubinsztein DC, Hon J, Stevens F *et al.* (1999) Apo E genotypes and risk of dementia in Down syndrome. *Am J Med Genet.* **88:** 344–7.

Sadovnick AD and Baird PA (1992) Life expectancy. In: SM Pueschel and JK Pueschel (eds) *Biomedical Concerns in Persons with Down Syndrome*. Paul H Brookes Publishing Co, Baltimore, MD.

Sadovnick AD, Yee IML and Hirst C (1994) The rate of the Down syndrome among offspring of women with Alzheimer disease. *Psychiatr Genet.* **4**: 87–9.

Saletu B (1991) EEG brain mapping in dementia and gerontopsychopharmacology. In: I Hindmarch, H Hippius and GK Wilcock (eds) *Dementia: molecules, methods and measures*. John Wiley & Sons Ltd, Chichester.

Sano M, Ernesto C, Thomas RG *et al.* (1997) A controlled trial of selegiline, alpha-tocopherol, or both as treatment for Alzheimer's disease. The Alzheimer's Disease Cooperative Study. *NEJM.* **336**: 1216–22.

Sattin RW (1992) Falls among older persons: a public health perspective. *Annu Rev Public Health.* **13**: 489–508.

Saunders AM, Hulette C and Welsh-Bohmer KA (1996) Specificity, sensitivity and predictive value of apolipoprotein-E genotyping for sporadic Alzheimer's disease. *Lancet.* **348**: 90–93.

Schapiro MB, Haxby JV, Grady CL *et al.* (1987) Quantitative CT analysis of brain morphometry in adult Down's syndrome at different ages. *Neurology.* **37**: 1424–47.

Schapiro MB, Ball MJ, Grady CL, Haxby JV, Kaye JA and Rapoport SI (1988) Dementia in Down's syndrome: cerebral glucose utilisation, neuropsychological assessment and neuropathology. *Neurology.* **38**: 938–42.

Schapiro MB, Haxby JV and Grady CL (1992) Nature of mental retardation and dementia in Down syndrome: study with PET, CT and neuropsychology. *Neurobiol Aging.* **13**: 723–34.

Scharre DW and Chang SI (2002) Cognitive and behavioral effects of quetiapine in Alzheimer disease patients. *Alzheimer Dis Assoc Disord.* **16**: 128–30.

Schatz RA (2003) Olanzapine for psychotic and behavioral disturbances in Alzheimer disease. *DICP.* **37**: 1321–4.

Schneider LS, Pollock VE and Lyness SA (1990) A meta-analysis of controlled trials of neuroleptic treatment in dementia. *J Am Geriatr Soc.* **38**: 553–63.

Schoenberg BS (1986) Epidemiology of dementia. *Neurol Clin.* **4**: 447–57.

Schoenberg BS, Kokmen E and Okazaki H (1987) Alzheimer's disease and other dementing illnesses in a defined United States population: incidence rates and clinical features. *Ann Neurol.* **22**: 724–9.

Schultz-Lampel D (2003) Bladder disorders in dementia and Alzheimer's disease. Ration diagnostic and therapeutic options. *Urologe Ausg.* **42**: 1579–87.

Schupf N (2002) Genetic and host factors for dementia in Down's syndrome. *Br J Psychiatry.* **180**: 405–10.

Schupf N and Sergievsky GH (2002) Genetic and host factors for dementia in Down's syndrome. *Br J Psychiatry.* **180**: 405–10.

Schupf N, Kapell D, Lee JE *et al.* (1996) Onset of dementia is associated with apolipoprotein E ε4. *Arch Neurol.* **40**: 799–801.

Schupf N, Kapell D, Nightingale B, Rodriguez A, Tyeko B and Mayeux R (1998) Earlier onset of Alzheimer's disease in men with Down syndrome. *Neurology.* **50**: 991–5.

Schupf N, Kapell D, Nightingale B *et al.* (2001a) Specificity of the five-fold increase in AD in mothers of adults with Down syndrome. *Neurology.* **57**: 979–84.

Schupf N, Patel B, Silverman W *et al.* (2001b) Elevated plasma amyloid beta-peptide 1–42 and onset of dementia in adults with Down syndrome. *Neurosci Lett.* **301**: 199–203.

Schupf N, Pang D, Patel BN *et al.* (2003) Onset of dementia is associated with age at menopause in women with Down's syndrome. *Ann Neurol.* **54**: 433–8.

Sekijima Y, Ikeda S, Tokuda T *et al.* (1998) Prevalence of dementia of Alzheimer type and apolipoprotein E phenotypes in aged patients with Down's syndrome. *Eur Neurol.* **39**: 234–7.

Seltzer GB, Schupf N and Wu HS (2001) A prospective study of menopause in women with Down's syndrome. *J Intellect Disabil Res.* **45**: 1–7.

Shulman R (1967) A survey of vitamin B$_{12}$ deficiency in an elderly psychiatric population. *Br J Psychiatry.* **113**: 241–51.

Sierpina VS, Wollschlaeger B and Blementhal M (2003) *Ginkgo biloba. Am Fam Physician.* **68**: 923–6.

Silverman W, Schupf N, Zigman W *et al.* (2004) Dementia in adults with mental retardation: assessment at a single point in time. *Am J Ment Retard.* **109**: 109–23.

Simard M and van Reekum R (2001) Dementia with Lewy bodies in Down's syndrome. *Int J Geriatr Psychiatry.* **16**: 311–20.

Skoog I and Gustafson D (2003) Hypertension, hypertension-clustering factors and Alzheimer's disease. *Neurol Res.* **25**: 675–80.

Slooter AJC, Houwing-Duistermaat JJ, Harskamp FV *et al.* (1999) Apolipoprotein E genotype and progression of Alzheimer's disease: the Rotterdam Study. *J Neurol.* **246**: 304–8.

Smith RP, Higuchi DA and Broze GJ (1990) Platelet coagulation factor XIa inhibitor, a form of Alzheimer's amyloid precursor protein. *Science.* **248**: 1126–8.

Soininen H, Partanen J, Jousmaki V *et al.* (1993) Age-related cognitive decline and electroencephalogram slowing in Down's syndrome as a model of Alzheimer's disease. *Neuroscience.* **53**: 57–63.

Spector A, Orrell M, Davies S and Woods B (2000a) *Reminiscence Therapy for Dementia.* Cochrane Database Systematic Reviews (4) CD001120. Update Software, Oxford.

Spector A, Orrell M, Davies S and Woods B (2000b) *Reality Orientation for Dementia.* Cochrane Database Systematic Reviews (4) CD001119. Update Softward, Oxford.

Steffelaar JW and Evenhuis HM (1989) Life expectancy, Down syndrome and dementia. *Lancet.* **1**: 492–3.

Strachan RW and Henderson JG (1967) Dementia and folate deficiency. *Q J Med.* **36**: 189–204.

Strittmatter WJ and Roses AD (1996) Apolipoprotein E and Alzheimer's disease. *Annu Rev Neurosci.* **19**: 53–77.

Strittmatter WJ, Saunders AM, Schmechel D, Pericak-Vance M and Enghild J (1993) Apolipoprotein E: high-avidity binding to beta-amyloid and increased frequency of type 4 allele in late-onset familial Alzheimer disease. *Proc Natl Acad Sci USA.* **90**: 1977–81.

Struwe F (1929) Histopathologische Untersuchungen uber Entstehung und Wesen der senilen plaques. *Z Neurol Psychiatrie.* **122**: 291–307.

Strydom A and Hassiotis A (2003) Diagnostic instruments for dementia in older people with intellectual disability in clinical practice. *Aging Ment Health.* **7**: 431–7.

Sulkava R, Wikstrom J, Aromaa A *et al.* (1985) Prevalence of severe dementia in Finland. *Neurology.* **35**: 1025–9.

Sung H, Hawkins BA, Eklund SJ *et al.* (1997) Depression and dementia in aging adults with Down syndrome: a case study approach. *Ment Retard.* **35**: 27–38.

Sylvester PE (1984) Ageing in the mentally retarded. In: J Dobbing, AD Clarke, JA Corbett, J Hogg and RO Robinson (eds) *Scientific Studies in Mental Retardation.* Royal Society of Medicine in association with Macmillan Press, London.

Sylvester PE (1986) The anterior commissure in Down's syndrome. *J Ment Defic Res.* **13**: 19–26.

Talbot C, Lendon C, Craddock N, Shears S, Morris JC and Goate A (1994) Protection against Alzheimer's disease with apoE E2. *Lancet.* **343**: 1432.

Tang MX, Jacobs D, Stern Y *et al.* (1996) Effect of oestrogen during menopause on risk and age at onset of Alzheimer's disease. *Lancet.* **348**: 429–32.

Tanzi RE, Gusella JF and Watkins PC (1987) Amyloid-protein gene: cDNA mRNA distribution, and genetic linkage near the Alzheimer locus. *Science.* **235**: 880–84.

Taphoorn MJ and Klein M (2004) Cognitive deficits in adult patients with brain tumours. *Lancet (Neurol.)* **3**: 159–68.

Tariot PN, Profenno LA and Ismail MS (2004) Efficacy of atypical antipsychotics in elderly patients with dementia. *J Clin Psychiatry.* **65**: 11–15.

Temple V, Jozsvai E, Konstantareas MM and Hewitt TA (2001) Alzheimer dementia in Down's syndrome: the relevance of cognitive ability. *J Intellect Disabil Res.* **45**: 47–55.

Teri L and Wagner A (1992) Alzheimer's disease and depression. *J Consult Clin Psychol.* **60**: 379–91.

Thase ME, Tigner R, Smeltzer D and Liss L (1984) Age-related neuropsychological deficits in Down's syndrome. *Biol Psychiatry.* **4**: 571–85.

Tierney MC, Fisher RH, Jewis AJ *et al.* (1988) The NINCDS–ADRDA work group criteria for the clinical diagnosis of probable Alzheimer's disease: a clinico-pathologic study of 57 cases. *Neurology.* **38**: 359–64.

Toran-Allerand CD, Miranda RC, Bentham WD *et al.* (1992) Estrogen receptors co-localize with low-affinity nerve growth factor receptors in cholinergic neurons of the basal forebrain. *Proc Natl Acad Sci USA.* **89**: 4668–72.

Treves T, Korczyn AD, Zilber N *et al.* (1986) Presenile dementia in Israel. *Arch Neurol.* **43**: 26–9.

Tsai MS, Tangalos EG, Petersen RC *et al.* (1994) Apolipoprotein E: risk factor for Alzheimer disease. *Am J Hum Genet.* **54**: 643–9.

Tsiouris JA and Patti PJ (1997) Drug treatment of depression associated with dementia or presented as 'pseudodementia' in older adults with Down syndrome. *J Appl Res Intellect Disabil.* **10**: 312–22.

Tune LE (1998) Depression and Alzheimer's disease. *Depression Anxiety.* **8**: 91–5.

Tyrrell PJ, Warrington EK, Frackowiak RSJ and Rossor MN (1990) Progressive degeneration of the right temporal lobe studied with positron emission tomography. *J Neurol Neurosurg Psychiatry.* **53**: 1046–50.

Tyrrell J, Cosgrave M, Hawi Z *et al.* (1998) A protective effect of apolipoprotein E e2 allele on dementia in Down's syndrome. *Soc Biol Psychiatry.* **43**: 397–400.

Tyrrell J, Cosgrave M, McPherson J *et al.* (1999) Presenilin 1 and alpha-1-antichymotrypsin polymorphisms in Down syndrome: no effect on the presence of dementia. *Am J Med Genet.* **8**: 616–20.

Tyrrell J, Cosgrave M, McCarron M *et al.* (2001) Dementia in people with Down's syndrome. *Int J Geriatr Psychiatry.* **16**: 1168–74.

Van Den Berg CM, Kazmi Y and Jann MW (2000) Cholinesterase inhibitors for the treatment of Alzheimer's disease in the elderly. *Drugs Aging.* **2**: 123–38.

Van Duijn CM, Stijnen T and Hofman A (1991) Risk factors for Alzheimer's disease: overview of the EURODEM collaborative re-analysis of case–control studies. EURODEM Risk Factors Research Group. *Int J Epidemiol.* **20 (Suppl. 2)**: S4–12.

Van Duijn CM, De Knijff P, Wehnert A *et al.* (1995) The apolipoprotein E epsilon 2 allele is associated with an increased risk of early-onset Alzheimer's disease and a reduced survival. *Ann Neurol.* **37**: 605–10.

Van Gool WA, Evenhuis HM and van Duijn CM (1995) A case–control study of apolipoprotein E genotypes in Alzheimer's disease associated with Down's syndrome. *Ann Neurol.* **38**: 225–30.

Van Nostrand WE, Schmaier AH, Farrow JS and Cunningham DD (1990) Protease nexin-II (amyloid beta protein precursor): a platelet alpha-granule protein. *Science.* **248**: 745–8.

Verhaart WJC and Jelgersma HC (1952) Early senile dementia in mongolian idiocy. Description of a case. *Folia Psychiatr Neerl.* **55**: 453–9.

Vieregge P, Ziemens G, Freudenberg M, Piosinski A, Muysers A and Schulze B (1991) Extrapyramidal features in advanced Down's syndrome: clinical evaluation and family history. *J Neurol Neurosurg Psychiatry.* **54**: 34–8.

Visser FE, Kuilman M, Oosting J, Overweg J, van Wijk J and van Huffelen AC (1996) Use of electroencephalography to detect Alzheimer's disease in Down's syndrome. *Acta Neurol Scand.* **94:** 97–103.

Visser SL, Stam FC, Van Tilburg W, Op den Velde W, Blom JL and De Rijke W (1976) Visual evoked response in senile and presenile dementia. *Electroencephalogr Clin Neurophysiol.* **40:** 385–92.

Vitiello MV and Borson S (2001) Sleep disturbances in patients with Alzheimer's disease: epidemiology, pathophysiology and treatment. *CNS Drugs.* **15:** 777–96.

Wang PN, Yang CL, Lin KN, Chen WT, Chwang LC and Lin HC (2004) Weight loss, nutritional status and physical activity in patients with Alzheimer's disease. A controlled study. *J Neurol.* **251:** 314–20.

Webber KM, Bowen R, Casadesus G, Perry G, Atwood CS and Smith MA (2004) Gonadotropins and Alzheimer's disease: the link between estrogen replacement therapy and neuroprotection. *Acta Neurobiol Exp.* **64:** 113–18.

Wechsler D (1974) *The Wechsler Intelligence Scale for Children – Revised.* Psychological Corporation, New York.

Weis S, Weber G, Neuhold A and Rett A (1991) Down syndrome: MR quantification of brain structures and comparison with normal control subjects. *Am J Neuroradiol.* **12:** 1207–11.

Wenger GC, Scott A and Seddon D (2002) The experience of caring for older people with dementia in a rural area: using services. *Aging Ment Health.* **6:** 30–38.

Wenk GL (2003) Neuropathological changes in Alzheimer's disease. *J Clin Psychiatry.* **64:** 7–10.

Whalley LJ (1982) The dementia of Down's syndrome and its relevance to etiological studies of Alzheimer's disease. *Ann N Y Acad Sci.* **396:** 39–53.

White H, Pieper C and Schmader K (1998) The association of weight change in Alzheimer's disease with severity of disease and mortality: a longitudinal analysis. *J Am Geriatr Soc.* **46:** 1223–7.

Whitehouse R, Chamberlain P and Tunna K (2000) Dementia in people with learning disability: a preliminary study into care staff knowledge and attributions. *Br J Learn Disabil.* **28:** 148–53.

Wilkinson H and Janicki MP (2002) The Edinburgh Principles with accompanying guidelines and recommendations. *J Intellect Disabil Res.* **46:** 279–84.

Williams PA, Jones GH and Briscoe M (1991) P300 and reaction-time measures in senile dementia of the Alzheimer type. *Br J Psychiatry.* **159:** 410–14.

Williams RS and Matthysse S (1986) Age-related changes in Down syndrome brain and the cellular pathology of Alzheimer Disease. *Prog Brain Res.* **70:** 49–67.

Wimo A, Winblad B, Stoffler A, Wirth Y and Mobius HJ (2003) Resource utilisation and cost analysis of memantine in patients with moderate to severe Alzheimer's disease. *Pharmacoeconomics.* **5:** 327–40.

Wisniewski KE, Wisniewski HM and Wen GY (1985) Occurrence of neuropathological changes and dementia of Alzheimer's disease in Down syndrome. *Ann Neurol.* **17:** 278–82.

Wisniewski T, Morelli L, Wegiel J, Levy E, Wisniewski HM and Frangione B (1995) The influence of apolipoprotein E isotypes on Alzheimer's disease pathology in 40 cases of Down's syndrome. *Ann Neurol.* **37:** 136–8.

Woods B (1998) Taking communication a step further? In: S Benson (ed.) *The Care Assistant's Guide to Working with People with Dementia.* Hawker Publications, London.

Wooltorton E (2002) Risperidone (Risperdal): increased incidence of cerebrovascular events in dementia trials. *Can Med Assoc J.* **167:** 1269–70.

Wooltorton E (2004) Olanzapine (Zyprexa): increased incidence of cerebrovascular events in dementia trials. *Can Med Assoc J.* **170:** 1395.

World Health Organization (1978) *Mental Disorders: glossary and guide to their classification in accordance with the Ninth Revision of the International Classification of Disease (ICD-9).* World Health Organization, Geneva.

World Health Organization (1992) *The ICD-10 Classification of Mental and Behavioural Disorders. Clinical descriptions and diagnostic guidelines.* World Health Organization, Geneva.

Yaffe K, Grady D, Pressman A and Cummings S (1998) Serum estrogen levels, cognitive performance, and risk of cognitive decline in older community women. *J Am Geriatr Soc.* **46:** 816–21.

Zigman WB, Schupf N, Sersen E and Silverman W (1996) Prevalence of dementia in adults with and without Down syndrome. *Am J Ment Retard.* **100:** 403–12.

Zigman W, Schupf N, Haveman M and Silverman W (1997) The epidemiology of Alzheimer disease in intellectual disability: results and recommendations from an international conference. *J Intellect Disabil Res.* **41:** 76–80.

Zigman WB, Schupf N, Urv T, Zigman A and Silverman W (2002) Incidence and temporal patterns of adaptive behavior change in adults with mental retardation. *Am J Ment Retard.* **107:** 161–74.

Zigman WB, Schupf N, Devenny DA *et al.* (2004) Incidence and prevalence of dementia in elderly adults with mental retardation without Down syndrome. *Am J Ment Retard.* **109:** 126–41.

Further sources of information

UK

Alzheimer's Society
Gordon House
10 Greencoat Place
London
SW1P 1PH
Tel: 020 7306 0606

Down's Syndrome Association
155 Mitcham Road
London
SW17 9PG
Tel: 0845 230 0372

MENCAP
123 Golders Lane
London
EC1Y ORT
Tel: 0207 454 0454

Carers UK
20–25 Glasshouse Yard
London
EC1A 4JT
Tel: 020 7490 8818

Scottish Down's Syndrome Association
158–160 Balgreen Road
Edinburgh
EH11 3AU
Tel: 0131 313 4225

Ireland

Down's Syndrome Ireland
41 Lower Dominick Street
Dublin 1
Ireland
Tel: 353 1873 0999

Rest of Europe

European Down Syndrome Association
Rue V Close, 41 B-4800
Polleur Verviers
Belgium
Tel: 3287 22335

USA

Administration on Developmental Disabilities
Department of Health and Human Services
Room 338-D, HHH Building
200 Independence Avenue, SW
Washington, DC 20201
Tel: (202) 690 6590

American Association on Mental Retardation
444 North Capitol Street, NW
Suite 846
Washington, DC 20001-1512
Tel: (202) 387 1968

National Down Syndrome Society
666 Broadway
New York, NY 10012-2317
Tel: (212) 416 9330

Useful websites

Alzheimer's Society (UK)
www.alzheimers.org.uk

Royal College of Psychiatrists (UK)
www.rcpsych.ac.uk

Down Syndrome Association (UK)
www.downs-syndrome.org.uk

National Down Syndrome Society
www.ndss.org

American Association on Mental Retardation
www.aamr.org

Administration on Developmental Disabilities
www.acf.dhhs.gov/programs/add

International Association for the Scientific Study of Intellectual Disabilities
www.iassid.org

List of Down syndrome internet sites
www.downsyndrome.com

Index